ABOUT THE AUTHOR

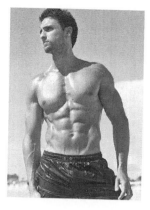

Hi,

I'm Mike and I've been training for over a decade now.

I believe that every person can achieve the body of his or her dreams, and I work hard to give everyone that chance by providing workable, proven advice grounded in science, not a desire to sell phony magazines, workout products, or supplements.

Through my work, I've helped thousands of people achieve their health and fitness goals, and I share everything I know in my books.

So if you're looking to get in shape and look great, then I think I can help you. I hope you enjoy my books and I'd love to hear from you at my site, www.muscleforlife.com.

Sincerely,
Mike

CONTENTS

THINNER
LEANER
STRONGER

THE SIMPLE SCIENCE OF BUILDING
THE ULTIMATE FEMALE BODY

Michael Matthews

oculus

This book is a general educational health-related information product and is intended for healthy adults, age 18 and over.

This book is solely for information and educational purposes and is not medical advice. Please consult a medical or health professional before you begin any exercise, nutrition, or supplementation program or if you have questions about your health.

There may be risks associated with participating in activities or using products mentioned in this book for people in poor health or with pre-existing physical or mental health conditions.

Because these risks exist, you will not use such products or participate in such activities if you are in poor health or have a pre-existing mental or physical health condition. If you choose to participate in these activities, you do so of your own free will and accord knowingly and voluntarily, assuming all risks associated with such activities.

Specific results mentioned in this book should be considered extraordinary and there are no "typical" results. As individuals differ, then results will differ.

Cover Designed by: Damon Freeman

Typesetting by Kiersten Lief

Published by Oculus Publishers.

www.oculuspublishers.com

Visit the author's website:

www.muscleforlife.com

THE PROMISE

No matter how bad you might think your genetics are, no matter how lost you might feel after trying and abandoning many types of workouts and diets, you absolutely, positively can have the lean, sexy body that you dream about.

WHAT IF I COULD SHOW you how to dramatically transform your body faster than you ever thought possible?

What if I gave you the exact formula of exercise and eating that makes losing 10 to 15 pounds of fat a breeze…and it only takes 8 to 12 weeks?

What if I showed you how to get a lean, toned physique that you love by investing *no more than 5 percent* of your time each day?

What if I told you that you can achieve that "Hollywood babe" body without having your life revolve around it—no long hours in the gym, no starving yourself, and no grueling cardio that turns your stomach. I'll even show you how to do it while still indulging in the "cheat" foods that you love every week like pasta, pizza, and ice cream.

And what if I promised to be at your side the entire way, helping you avoid the scams, pitfalls, and problems that most women fall into, helping you systematically achieve the body of your dreams, and basically doing everything I can to see you get into the best shape of your life?

Imagine if you got up every morning, looked in the mirror, and couldn't help but smile at your reflection. Imagine the boost in confidence you'd feel if you didn't have that belly or thigh fat anymore, or if you were no longer "just another woman," but instead had lean, sexy curves and were "that hot chick."

Imagine, just 12 weeks from now, being constantly complimented on how you look and asked what the *heck* you're doing to make such startling gains. Imagine enjoying the added benefits of high energy levels, no aches and pains, better spirits, and knowing that you're getting healthier every day.

Well, you *can* have all of these things, and it's not *nearly* as complicated as the fitness industry wants you to believe (more on that in a minute). It doesn't matter if you're twenty-one or sixty-one, in shape or completely not. No matter who you are, I promise you: you *can* change your body into whatever you desire.

And last but not least, maybe there's a part of you that wouldn't mind showing us guys how it's done—how to train properly, how to eat properly, and how to look amazing. Well, you can totally be that woman.

So, would you like my help?

If you answered "Yes!" then you've taken a *leap*, not a step, toward your goals to become a leaner, more shaped and sculpted you.

Your journey to the ultimate female body begins as soon as you turn to the next page.

INTRODUCTION

WHY *THINNER LEANER STRONGER* IS DIFFERENT

I'M GOING TO TELL YOU something that the kings of the multi-billion dollar health and fitness industry don't want you to know: You don't need any of their crap to get into shape and to look better than you ever have before.

- You don't need to starve yourself with super low-calorie diets to lose weight and keep it off. In fact, this is how you ruin your metabolism and ensure that any weight lost will come back with a *vengeance.*

- You don't need to spend hundreds of dollars per month on worthless supplements or fat loss pills.

- You don't need to constantly change up your exercise routines to "confuse" your muscles. I'm pretty sure that muscles lack cognitive abilities, so this approach is a good way to just confuse you instead.

- You don't need to grind out hours and hours of boring cardio to shed ugly belly fat and love handles and get lean and toned. (How many flabby treadmillers have you come across over the years?)

- You don't need to completely abstain from "cheat" foods while losing weight or maintaining your ideal physique. If you plan cheat meals correctly, you can actually *accelerate* fat loss.

These are just a small sampling of the harmful fallacies commonly believed by many women, and they will bury you in a rut of frustration, deliver little to no results, and inevitably lead to quitting.

That was actually my motivation for creating *Thinner Leaner Stronger*: For many years now, I've had friends, family, acquaintances, and co-workers approach me for fitness advice, and they were almost always convinced of many strange, unworkable ideas about diet and exercise.

By educating them in the same way as I'm about to educate you, I've helped people melt away fat, build lean, attractive muscle, and not only look great, but feel great too. And, while helping friends, friends of friends, and family is fulfilling, I want to be able to help thousands (or tens or even hundreds of thousands!). Thus, *Thinner Leaner Stronger* was born.

Now, where did the many fitness and nutrition myths come from? Well, I don't want to waste your time with the boring history of the world of exercise, supplements, and information resources, but the long story short is simply this:

When people are willing to spend big amounts of money on certain types of products or to solve specific problems, there will never be a scarcity of new, "cutting edge" things for them to empty their wallets on, and there will always be scores of brilliant marketers inventing new schemes to keep people spending.

It's pretty simple, really. All we have to do is look where most people get their training and nutritional advice from. Almost everyone gets it from one or more of these three sources: magazines, personal trainers, or friends. The fact is you'll almost never learn anything useful from any of them.

How can I make such bold claims, you wonder? Because I've seen it all, tried it all, and while I don't know it all, I do know what works and what doesn't.

THE NOT-SO-SECRET AGENDA OF MOST FITNESS MAGAZINES

The primary goal of most fitness magazines is to sell supplements for the companies controlling them, and they work *damn* well. The magazines push products in various ways. They have pretty advertisements all over the place, they regularly run "advertorials" (advertisements disguised as informative articles), and they balance the lot of sales pitches with some actual articles that provide workout and nutrition advice (which also, in many cases, end with product recommendations of some kind).

So, this is the first blow that magazines deal to you: They give you a lot of "advice" that is geared first and foremost to selling you products, not helping you achieve your goals.

The supplement companies know that if they can just keep getting these magazines into people's hands, they will keep selling products. So, how do they ensure that you will keep buying? By coming up with a constant flow of new advice and ideas, of course.

And this is the second, probably more harmful, blow: They inundate you with all kinds of false ideas about what it takes to get into great shape. If they told the simple truth every month, they would have maybe 20 articles or so that they could re-print over and over. Instead, they get quite creative with all kinds of sophisticated (but useless) workout routines, "tricks," and diets (that include certain supplements to really MAXIMIZE the effectiveness, of course).

The bottom line is that you can't trust these types of magazines. They are all either owned by or financially dependent upon supplement companies, and what I outlined above is the game they play.

MOST PERSONAL TRAINERS ARE JUST A WASTE OF MONEY... END OF STORY

Most personal trainers are a waste of time and money.

Every week I see trainers who either have no clue what they're doing or who just don't care about their clients. These poor people are paying $50-$75 per hour to do silly, ineffective workout routines that usually consist of the wrong exercises done with bad form (and they make little or no gains).

And, let's not forget that many personal trainers aren't even in good shape themselves, which always confuses me. How can you honestly sell yourself as a fitness expert when you're flabby and out of shape? Who could possibly believe you? Well, for some reason, these types of trainers get business all the time, and their clients almost always stay flabby and out of shape themselves.

To compound the disservice, most trainers don't even bother giving their clients nutritional plans, which *really* ensures lackluster gains. The fact is that 70-80% of how you look is a reflection of how you eat. Fat, skinny, toned, whatever—exercise is only 20-30% of the equation. Eat wrong, and you will stay fat no matter how much cardio you do; eat wrong, and you will stay skinny and weak no matter how much you struggle with weights. Eat right, however, and you can unlock the maximum potential gains from working out: rapid, long-term fat loss and lean, sexy muscle that will turn heads and get your friends and family talking.

You might be wondering why these trainers know so little as certified professionals. Well, I have several good friends who are trainers, and they've all told me the same thing, which is that passing the certification test does *not* make you an expert—it means that you can memorize some basic information about nutrition and exercise…that's about it.

While some people are happy to pay a trainer just to force themselves to show up every day, trainers are usually in a similar boat as the magazines. They have to constantly justify their existence, and they do it by changing up routines and talking about "sophisticated" workout principles (that they read about in the magazines)…and when it's all said and done, their clients waste thousands of dollars to make little progress.

That said, there absolutely *are* great trainers out there who are in awesome shape themselves, who *do* know how to quickly and effectively get others into shape, and who do really care. If you're one of them and you're reading this book, I applaud you because you're carrying the weight of the entire profession on your shoulders.

THE "SECRET" OF SOME OF THE HOTTEST WOMEN IN THE WORLD

If I say "hottest women in the world," what immediately comes to mind?

Chances are you thought of Victoria's Secret models. While it's trendy for celebrities to pretend their bodies come effortlessly, don't fall for it—these woman work hard to achieve their enviable physiques.

But here's something many women don't know: Victoria's Secret models train a lot like guys. What do I mean? Sure, they do cardio, but they rely primarily on *weight training* to look the way they do—to have toned, sexy arms; thin, defined legs; and a perfectly shaped butt.

Don't believe me?

Miranda Kerr lifts weights four days per week, and relies on exercises like the Barbell Squat, Barbell Lunge, and Barbell Reverse Lunge to lift her butt and tone her legs.

Chanel Iman said she has trouble toning her body and relies on "a lot of squats and weight lifting" to keep her body in runway shape.

Alessandra Ambrosio squats, lunges, and deadlifts for her famous butt and legs.

I could go on but you get the point.

Now, this might leave you a little confused. "Doesn't weight training lead to bulky, ugly muscles?" you might be wondering.

Well, that's one of the Big Lies in the world of women's fitness. Building muscle is the key to accelerating your metabolism, getting sexy curves, and staying lean.

You see, women don't build muscle like guys do. You have approximately one *sixteenth* of the testosterone of the average guy, and testosterone is the primary driving force behind muscle growth.

What this means is that it's basically impossible for you to bulk up in the same way as us guys. Bigger and strong muscles on a woman looks very different than on a guy.

The scary women that walk the stages of bodybuilding shows are training harder than you can imagine, and are on more drugs than you can imagine (steroids, among others) to look that way.

For the normal woman, moderate and proper weight training is actually the key to getting thin, lean, toned, and strong.

WHAT *THINNER LEANER STRONGER* IS ALL ABOUT

I don't know about you, but I don't exercise to have fun or hang out with friends—I exercise to look and feel better, and I want to get the most from my efforts. If I can get better results by working out half as long as the other person, that's what I want to do. If my options are to shed ten pounds of fat in a month by doing the same "boring" routine every week or to squeak out two pounds of fat loss by doing the latest dynamic inertia muscle confusion routine, I'll choose the former.

Thinner Leaner Stronger is all about exercising and eating properly and getting results. It gives you a precise training and nutrition regimen that delivers maximum gains in the least amount of time. The exercises are nothing new and sophisticated, but you've probably never approached them like how I'm going to teach you. There's nothing cutting edge or complicated about how to eat correctly, but most people have it all wrong.

With *Thinner Leaner Stronger*, you can lose ten to fifteen pounds of fat in your first three months of following the program. That's a pretty drastic change. People are going to start asking you for workout advice.

If you don't need to lose weight but are naturally skinny and are looking to tone up and create some definition in your arms, legs, abs, and butt, *Thinner Leaner Stronger* will show you exactly how to do it (and it has everything to do with making your muscles bigger and stronger, but not in the same way as us guys!).

So, are you ready? Great.

Here's the first step: *Forget what you think you know about working out.* I know, it might sound a little harsh, but trust me—it's for your own good. Just let it all go, approaching *Thinner Leaner Stronger* with an open mind.

Along the way, you'll find that certain things you believed or did were right while others were wrong, and that's okay. Just follow the program exactly as I lay it out, and then let the results speak for themselves. If you do, I can guarantee that you'll never go looking for another fitness plan ever again.

So, let's get started!

1

THE HIDDEN BARRIER TO ACHIEVING YOUR FITNESS AND HEALTH GOALS

YOU MAY HAVE WONDERED WHY so many people are utterly confused on the subjects of health and fitness. Ask around one day, and you're liable to receive all kinds of conflicting, illogical advice and opinions.

Counting calories doesn't work. Broccoli has more protein than chicken. Any carbs you eat at night will automatically turn into body fat. If you eat fats, you'll get fat (and its corollary: eat little-to-no fat to lose fat). You have to eat a lot of small meals every day to lose weight.

I've actually been told all of these things. Pretty scary, right?

So how does this happen? Why are people so susceptible to false information, lies, and weird ideas?

While that question might sound like it has a deep, philosophical answer, it's pretty simple, really.

The next time you hear someone saying that counting calories isn't necessary or doesn't work, ask them this simple question:

What is a calorie?

One for one, they will just stand there with a confused look on their faces. They don't have a clue what the word means. And that's only the beginning, of course.

What is a carbohydrate?

What is protein?

What is fat?

What is muscle?

What is a hormone?

What is a vitamin?

What is an amino acid?

Very few people can actually define these words, so of course they can't understand the subject and will believe nearly anything they're told. How can you gain a full and proper understanding of a subject when you don't understand the words used to explain it?

Well, that's why *words* are the biggest hidden barrier to understanding that almost everyone completely overlooks.

Simply put, if you have misunderstandings about the words being used to communicate specific concepts, you will not duplicate the communications exactly—you will reach your own distorted conclusions due to misinterpretation. If I were to tell you, "The children have to leave at crepuscule," you might wonder what I am talking about. "Crepuscule" simply means the time of the day when the sun is just below the horizon, especially the period between sunset and dark. The sentence now makes sense, doesn't it?

In school, many of us were taught to simply guess at the meanings of words by looking at the surrounding context or by comparing the word to other words in our vocabularies. This is, of course, a very unreliable method of study because the person writing the text had a specific concept to communicate and chose exact words based on specific understandings. If you want to receive the information in the same light, you must share the same understanding of the words used to convey it, not come to subjective understandings based on what you think the words might mean.

With "crepuscule" in the example above, context only reveals that the word must be a time of day, which isn't enough information to guess the word. Then, you're left with looking at the word itself, maybe thinking, "Well, 'crepuscule' looks like 'crepes,' which are often eaten in the morning, so I guess it means 'after breakfast'?"

That's why the first part of *Thinner Leaner Stronger* is clarifying the key words that will be used throughout the book. I know that reading the definitions of words is kind of dry and unsexy, but trust me, it will help *a lot*. It's the only way you can be sure that we're on the same page and that you're understanding things the way I mean you to.

I took care in putting together these key word lists to build your understanding from the simple to the more complex, and I think you'll find the learning curve very mild. I'm sure you will breeze right through it and have quite a few light bulbs turn on.

By the end of the next few chapters of this book, you will know more about health, nutrition, and fitness than most everyone you know. It's really that bad out there.

So let's get started with the first list of key words.

2

WHAT MOST PEOPLE DON'T KNOW ABOUT HEALTH, NUTRITION, AND FITNESS

PART ONE: SCIENCE OF THE BODY

ENERGY: 1. *Energy* is the power received from electricity, fuel, food, and other sources in order to work or produce motion.

2. *Energy* is the physical or mental strength of a person that can be directed toward some activity.

CHEMISTRY: *Chemistry* is the branch of science that deals with the identification of the substances that matter is composed of, the study of their characteristics, and the ways that they interact, combine, and change.

CHEMICAL: 1. *Chemical* means having to do with chemistry, or how substances are made up and the reactions and changes they go through.

2. A *chemical* is any substance that can undergo a chemical process or change.

Note: Usually when people say *chemicals*, they are referring to man-made substances, but the definition isn't limited to just this.

ORGANISM: An *organism* is a single living thing, such as a person, animal, or plant.

CELL: A *cell* is the basic unit of all living organisms. Some living organisms exist only as a single cell. An average-size man contains 60 to 100 trillion cells. Cells keep themselves alive, produce energy, exchange information with neighboring cells, multiply, and eventually die when their time has come. Each cell is a small container of chemicals and water wrapped up by a thin sheet of material.

TISSUE: *Tissue* is body material in animals and plants that's made up of large numbers of cells that are similar in form and function.

MUSCLE: *Muscles* are masses of tissue in the body, often attached to bones, that can tighten and relax to produce movement.

FAT: 1. *Fat* is naturally oily or greasy extra flesh in the body kept under the skin.

2. *Fat* is a substance of this type made from plant products that's used in cooking. Some fats are important nutrients for the body to use in building cells and accomplishing other bodily activities.

ORGAN: An *organ* is a part of an organism that's made of a group of two or more tissues that work together to achieve a specific function.

Note: Muscle is not an *organ* because a muscle is just one kind of tissue, and an *organ* must consist of at least two kinds of *tissue* to be considered an organ.

GRAM: A *gram* is a unit of weight in the metric system. One pound is about 454 grams.

KILOGRAM: A *kilogram* is equal to a thousand grams. There are a little more than two pounds to every kilogram.

MILLIGRAM: A *milligram* is one thousandth of a gram. There are one thousand *milligrams* in a gram.

CELSIUS: *Celsius* is a scale of temperature on which water freezes at 0 degrees and boils at 100 degrees.

Note: In the Fahrenheit scale used in the U.S., water freezes at 32 degrees and boils at 212 degrees.

CALORIE: A *calorie* is a measurement unit of the amount of energy that can be produced by food. One *calorie* is enough energy to raise the temperature of one gram of water by one degree Celsius.

Thus, when you're referring to the calories contained in food, you're referring to the potential energy stored in the food.

Note: Extra *calories* taken into the body beyond what is needed to run the body or build muscle can be stored as fat.

NUTRIENT: A *nutrient* is a substance that gives a living body something that it needs to live and grow.

FOOD: *Food* is material taken into the body to provide it with the nutrients it needs for energy and growth. Food is fuel for the body.

MATTER: *Matter* is any material in the universe that has mass and size.

ELEMENT: An *element* (also called a *chemical element*) is a substance that cannot be broken down into smaller parts by a chemical reaction. There are over 100 elements and they are the primary building blocks of matter.

COMPOUND: A *compound* is a substance made up of two or more different elements.

BREAK DOWN: To *break* something *down* means to separate it into smaller, more basic parts.

MOLECULE: A *molecule* is the smallest particle of any compound that still exists as that substance. If you were to break it down any further, it would separate into the elements that make it up (meaning it would no longer exist as that original substance).

ACID: An *acid* is a chemical compound that usually eats away at materials and often tastes sour.

PROTEIN: *Proteins* are naturally occurring compounds that are used for growth and repair in the body and to build cells and tissues. Muscle tissue contains lots of *protein*. *Protein* keeps you strong and makes your bones last. It is an essential nutrient for life.

AMINO ACID: *Amino acids* are very small units of material that protein is built out of.

GAS: A *gas* is a substance that is in an air-like form (not solid or liquid).

CARBON: *Carbon* is a common non-metallic chemical element that is found in much of the matter on earth and in all life.

OXYGEN: *Oxygen* is a chemical element that is a gas with no color or smell and is necessary for most living things to survive.

HYDROGEN: *Hydrogen* is a colorless, odorless gas that is very flammable and is the simplest and most abundant chemical element in the universe.

CARBOHYDRATE: *Carbohydrates* are molecules composed of carbon, oxygen, and hydrogen. *Carbohydrates* are important nutrients for energy and for building cells in the body. The word *carbohydrate* is formed by *carbo-* which means *carbon*, and *-hydrate* which means *water*.

DIGESTION: *Digestion* is the process of breaking down food so that it can be absorbed and used by the body.

ENZYME: An *enzyme* is a substance produced by organisms that helps cause specific chemical reactions.

METABOLISM: *Metabolism* is the term for the series of processes by which molecules from food are broken down to release energy, which is then used to fuel the cells in the body and to create more complex molecules used for building new cells. *Metabolism* is necessary for life and is how the body creates and maintains the cells that make it up.

ANABOLISM: *Anabolism* is a metabolic process in which energy is used to make more complex substances (such as tissue) from simpler ones.

CATABOLISM: *Catabolism* is the production of energy through the conversion of complex molecules (such as muscle or fat) into simpler ones.

3

WHAT MOST PEOPLE DON'T KNOW ABOUT HEALTH, NUTRITION, AND FITNESS
PART TWO: NUTRITION

HEALTH: 1. A person's *health* is the general condition of his/her body or mind, especially in regards to strength and energy as well as the presence or lack of disease.

2. *Health* is the state of being well; free of any illnesses or injuries.

HEALTHY: Being *healthy* means that you are in a good condition physically with good strength and energy levels and free from illness or damage.

NOURISH: To *nourish* is to provide something with the substances needed to grow, live, and be healthy.

NUTRIENT: A *nutrient* is a substance that provides nourishment essential for life and growth.

NUTRITION: *Nutrition* is the process of getting nourishment, especially the process of getting food and nutrients and utilizing them to stay healthy, grow, and build and replace tissues.

DIET: 1. One's *diet* is the food and drink that he or she usually consumes.

2. A *diet* is a special course of controlled or restricted intake of food or drink for a particular purpose, such as losing weight, supporting exercise, or for medical maintenance.

SUGAR: *Sugar* is a class of sweet-tasting carbohydrates that come from various plants, fruits, honey, and other sources.

SUCROSE: *Sucrose* is the kind of sugar most commonly called "table sugar." It is usually in the form of a white powder and is used as a sweetener.

It is most often taken from natural sources but can be made artificially as well.

GLUCOSE: *Glucose* is a very simple sugar that is an important energy source in living things. Most carbohydrates are broken down in the body into glucose, which is the main source of fuel for all cells.

GLYCOGEN: *Glycogen* is a substance found in bodily tissues that acts as a store of carbohydrates.

Note: When the body has extra glucose, it stores it in the liver and muscles, and this stored form of glucose is called *glycogen*. Glycogen is like the body's back-up fuel, and it releases glucose into the bloodstream when the body needs a quick energy boost. It doesn't matter whether you eat lettuce or candy; both end up as glucose in the body. The only difference is that the lettuce takes a lot longer to break down into glucose than the sugary candy. (The different effects of each will be described in detail in Chapter 17.)

BLOOD SUGAR: Your *blood sugar* level is the amount of glucose in your blood. Glucose is carried in the blood and delivered to cells so that it can be broken down and the energy can be stored or used.

SIMPLE CARBOHYDRATE: A *simple carbohydrate* is a very simple form of sugar that is usually sweet tasting and is broken down into glucose very quickly.

COMPLEX CARBOHYDRATE: A *complex carbohydrate* is a carbohydrate that is made up of many molecules of "simple carbohydrates" linked together. Because of this, it takes the body longer to break it down into glucose.

STARCH: *Starch* is a complex carbohydrate that is found naturally in many fruits and vegetables and is sometimes added to other foods to thicken them. In its pure form it is a white powder. Although starch is a complex carbohydrate, some particular foods high in starch break down into glucose quickly, like a simple carbohydrate would.

HORMONE: A *hormone* is a chemical made in the body that gets transported by the blood or other bodily fluids to cells and organs to cause some action or to have a specific effect.

INSULIN: *Insulin* is a hormone that consists of protein and is made in the organ known as the pancreas. When you eat food, your body breaks it down into nutrients that are then released into the bloodstream. The body also produces *insulin*, which causes muscles, organs, and fat tissue to take up the nutrients and either use them or store them as body fat.

INDEX: An *index* is a system of listing information in an order that allows one to easily compare it to other information.

GLYCEMIC INDEX: The *glycemic index* (or *GI*) is a scale that measures the effect of different carbohydrates on one's blood sugar level. Carbohydrates that break down slowly and release glucose into the blood slowly are low on the *glycemic index*. Carbohydrates that break down quickly will release glucose into the blood quickly, causing insulin levels to suddenly spike; these are high on the *glycemic index*. Below 55 on the *GI* is considered low, and above 70 is considered high. Pure glucose is 100 on the *GI*.

GRAIN: *Grains* are seeds of different kinds of grass that are used for many kinds of food. *Grains* are often ground up into a powder called flour.

WHEAT: *Wheat* is a plant that produces grain. It's commonly used for making bread and pasta.

WHITE BREAD: *White bread* is bread made from wheat flour that has had parts of the grains removed and has been bleached in order for it to bake easier and last longer.

Note: Most of the nutrients are removed or killed in the process of making white bread, turning the bread into a simpler carbohydrate.

WHOLE GRAIN: Foods containing grains that have not had parts removed are called *whole grain* foods. *Whole grain* bread is a source of complex carbohydrates, oils, fats, and some protein.

FIBER: *Fiber* is a substance found in some grains, fruit, and vegetables that cannot be digested. *Fiber* serves to soak up extra water and push other food through the digestive system. It helps push useless food waste out of the body, preventing it from sitting in the system and clogging it. *Fiber* is considered to play a role in the prevention of many diseases of the digestive tract.

FATTY ACIDS: *Fatty acids* are the molecules that make up fat cells. Some *fatty acids* are needed for building parts of cells and tissues in the body. *Fatty acids* contain twice as many calories as carbohydrates and proteins and are mainly used to store energy in fat tissue.

OIL: *Oil* is fat that is in a liquid form at room temperature. *Oil* has a slippery feeling and does not mix well with water.

ESSENTIAL FATTY ACIDS: Some fatty acids are called *essential fatty acids* because they are needed for many important bodily functions. They are received from the oils of some plants and fish.

4

WHAT MOST PEOPLE DON'T KNOW ABOUT HEALTH, NUTRITION, AND FITNESS
PART THREE: HEALTH

SUPPLEMENT: A *supplement* is a quantity of any substance that's added to fill in a deficiency or make something more complete.

DIETARY SUPPLEMENT: A *dietary* (or nutritional) *supplement* is a product taken to give a person nutrients that are not contained in a large enough quantity in the person's diet.

VITAMIN: A *vitamin* is a naturally occurring compound that is needed in small amounts by the body but cannot be produced in the body, and therefore, it needs to be absorbed from an outside source. Not getting enough *vitamins* in your diet leads to many undesirable conditions and possibly fatal diseases.

MINERAL: A *mineral* is a compound that is found in non-living matter. They are not naturally created inside of living organisms, but they are required by the body to maintain proper function.

DEHYDRATION: The human body is made of 75% water. Water is lost by sweating, urination, and breathing, and this water needs to be replaced every day. When not enough water has been replaced for the body to properly function, it is called *dehydration*. This gives you a headache, makes you tired and weak, and if not fixed, can be fatal since all vital organs need water to exist and function.

NERVE: A *nerve* is a bundle of fibers in the body that carries electrical messages between the brain, spinal cord, organs, and muscles. These messages give sensations and cause muscles and organs to operate. Nerves are the communication system of the body.

SALT: *Salt* is a mineral that is used a lot in cooking for seasoning food. It has its own taste that is one of the basic tastes of the human diet. *Salt* is a very important electrolyte and mineral that is necessary for many bodily functions.

PROCESSED: To *process* food means to use chemicals or a machine to change or preserve the food.

Note: The action of *processing* foods done by food manufacturers often kills many of the vitamins, minerals, and other nutrients that the body needs, and it typically adds chemicals into the food that are harmful to the body. *Processed* food usually has many more calories than it would otherwise have, but without the nutrients that usually go along with it.

ORGANIC: *Organic* food is food that has been raised and made with very little or no use of artificially made chemical pesticides and fertilizers, according to a standard now regulated by the government. With the current standards in the U.S., foods that have ingredients that are at least 95% organic and that have been prepared with very low or no artificial chemicals added or used in processing can be sold with the label *organic.*

ALL NATURAL: *Natural* foods are foods that have gone through very little or no processing. Some people like to eat *all natural* foods to avoid artificial, added chemicals and "empty calories."

Note: *All natural* foods have not been heavily processed, but that does not mean that they are organic. *All natural* labels can be used more freely and are not as strictly regulated as organic foods. *All natural* foods have usually had chemical fertilizers and pesticides used on them unless they are also marked as organic.

CHOLESTEROL: *Cholesterol* is a soft, waxy substance found among some fats that moves through your bloodstream and into your body's cells. Your body makes some *cholesterol,* and the rest comes from animal products consumed, such as meat, fish, eggs, butter, cheese, and whole milk. *Cholesterol* is not found in foods made from plants.

Note: One kind of *cholesterol,* known as *"good cholesterol,"* is necessary for survival and is used in building the cells in the body and for other important functions. *"Bad cholesterol"* can get stuck in your bloodstream and block the flow of blood, causing a heart attack if you have too much of it in the bloodstream.

BODY MASS INDEX (BMI): The *Body Mass Index* (*BMI*) is a scale that uses a system of numbers for estimating about how much a person should weigh depending on how tall he or she is. The *BMI* is meant to give a vague estimate for large groups of people or whole populations. When the *BMI* is used for evaluating an individual, it is very often inaccurate because of different body types, like having a thin frame, a lot of muscle tissue, or being very tall.

PERCENTAGE: A *percent*, or *percentage*, is a way of expressing a number as a fraction of 100. *Percent* means "for every hundred," so 50% means half because 50 is half of 100.

BODY FAT PERCENTAGE: Your *body fat percentage* is a measurement of the amount of fat that you have in your body expressed as a percentage of your total body weight. This is a more precise measurement of fat than the BMI as it directly measures the person's fat no matter what that person's body type is or how much weight in muscle that person has, which are not taken into account on the BMI.

Note: The amount of fat your body needs to accomplish basic body functions for living is about 2-4% body fat in men and 10-12% in women.

OVERWEIGHT: Being *overweight* means that a person has more fat than is considered to be healthy.

OBESE: Someone who is *obese* has so much extra fat that it is extremely likely to have bad effects on that person's health and can lead to many diseases. Being *obese* is determined by being over 30 on the BMI, or by having more than 32% body fat in women, and 25% in men.

5

THE 8 BIGGEST MUSCLE BUILDING MYTHS & MISTAKES

NINE OUT OF TEN PEOPLE you see in the gym lifting weights don't train correctly. In many cases, I wouldn't even bother getting out of bed in the morning to do their training routines.

They're usually following programs they found in magazines or on the internet, or maybe they got them from friends or trainers. They are stuck in a rut of no gains or eking out slow, stubborn gains.

Most people also compound their training mistakes by eating incorrectly—they're eating too much, eating too little, not getting the right amounts and types of macronutrients, and are making other various muscle-robbing mistakes.

So, I'd like to take a moment here to address the eight most common myths and mistakes of gaining lean muscle, as this will be an important part of building your dream body.

Chances are good that you have fallen victim to one or more of these fallacies at some point in the past (and if you haven't, it's probably because you're brand new, which actually gives you a great advantage: You get to do it right from day one!).

MYTH & MISTAKE #1:
THE LIES OF TONING AND SHAPING

Most weight training advice for women revolves around three goals: toning, shaping, and sculpting.

"Toning" generally refers to making your muscles "tighter" when you aren't flexing them.

"Shaping" generally refers to actually changing the shape of your muscles, such as making your butt rounder.

"Sculpting" generally refers to building a muscle while reducing body fat so it actually shows, and this is the most useful of the three terms (and I'll explain why).

Most books and magazines for women recommend doing a ton of repetitions with light weights to tone muscle "without making it bigger." This is a myth. If you don't use enough weight to challenge your muscles, they won't grow. If they don't grow, they won't look any better than they currently do, even if you lost a bunch of weight. This is why many woman look "skinny fat"—they don't have much fat on their body, but they don't have any muscle to speak of, either.

The simple fact of the matter is without well-trained muscles, your body will never look the way you want, no matter how little fat you're carrying.

While it helps sell magazines, there's no way to change the shape of your muscles. You can make them bigger and stronger, which can result in a more aesthetic shape for a leg or arm, but your genetics will determine the actual shape of the leg or arm.

The claims that certain forms of strength training will make "long, lean" muscles like a dancer's while others will result in "bulky, ugly" muscles like a she-male are bogus. Whether you do Pilates, yoga, or weight training to strengthen and build your muscles, their shape will come out the same, with the difference being that weight training will grow your muscles faster than Pilates or yoga (and yoga and Pilates offer things that weight training doesn't, of course, such as flexibility, intense sweating, inner calm, etc.).

Now, with that being said, you can absolutely have a great butt, shapely legs, and sexy arms. But you can't necessarily have the same butt as your favorite model or celebrity as you could both do the same exercises and be equally lean, and your butts will be shaped differently.

"Sculpting" best describes what is actually possible. You can build your muscles and reduce your body fat percentage, which will give you that thin, athletic "beach body" that so many women envy. That's what this book is all about.

MYTH & MISTAKE #2:
LIFTING WEIGHTS WILL MAKE YOU BULKY

I know I've already address this earlier, but I really want to drive it home.

The bottom line is muscle is really hard to build, even for us guys. Never once has a guy walked into a gym worried about getting too big that day. Why not? Because any guy that trains naturally knows how tough it is to gain each and every pound of muscle. We have to train hard and eat right every day, and it takes years to go from "normal" to anything resembling a cover model.

Women have it way harder in this regard. Way, way harder. So hard, in fact, that I will say this:

Unless you're a genetic freak, you not only won't get bulky from weight training, you couldn't even if you wanted to.

Your body simply can't do it. It lacks the hormones and genetic programming.

In fact, you'll be lucky to gain ten pounds of muscles in your first six months of following my program. But don't worry—gaining this kind of weight will be exactly what you want. Adding muscle weight means a tighter body and stronger metabolism.

MYTH & MISTAKE #3:
THE MORE YOU EXERCISE, THE BETTER

I don't know about you, but I hate long workouts. Who wants to spend two hours in a gym every day? Only the over-zealous newbies who think that the grueling seventeenth set is where the magic happens, or the obsessed meatheads who like to squat until their noses bleed and deadlift until they puke (yes, these guys are out there).

The fact is, exercising for too long each day can actually lead to *overtraining*, which not only robs you of muscle growth and fat loss and makes you feel run-down and lethargic, but can actually cause you to *lose* muscle and *hold onto* fat.

Yes, that's right—a couple hours of intense weight or resistance training can actually make you less toned and weaker. You are simply breaking down the muscle too much for your body to repair it optimally. Of course you don't want to under-train either by doing too little, which is why *Thinner Leaner Stronger* weight workouts are built to achieve the maximum muscle stimulation that your body can efficiently repair.

More sets also means more time spent working out, of course, and this too is detrimental to your gains. As you exercise, your body releases hormones such as testosterone and growth hormone, and both are conducive to muscle growth and fat loss. In response to the physical stress, however, your body also releases a hormone called *cortisol*. This hormone helps increase blood sugar levels and fight inflammation, but it also interferes with your body's ability to use protein correctly and stops muscle growth. Acute cortisol spikes while training are good and have been shown to improve the body's ability to build muscle[1] (and, incidentally, research has shown that training in the range of 75% of one rep max leads to more cortisol production than training with lower weights[2]), but if your levels remain elevated for too long, it becomes a problem. One of the best ways to control cortisol is to *keep your training sessions short.*

The bottom line is that if your exercise program is built correctly, you can achieve stunning gains by training for no longer than 45 to 60 minutes per day.

MYTH & MISTAKE #4:
YOU HAVE TO "FEEL THE BURN" TO GET BIGGER AND STRONGER MUSCLES

How many times have you heard people yelling for each other to "Make it burn!" and "Get another three reps!"? They think that pumping out reps until the stinging pain is unbearable causes maximum growth. "No pain, no gain," right? Wrong. This is probably one of the worst fallacies out there: that muscle "burn" and pump are paramount in achieving growth. Well, they aren't.

When your muscles are burning, what you're actually feeling is a build-up of lactic acid in the muscle, which builds as you contract your muscles again and again. Lactic acid does trigger what's known as the "anabolic cascade," which is a cocktail of growth-inducing hormones, but elevating lactic acid levels higher and higher doesn't mean you build more and more muscle.

When people spend a couple of hours in the gym pounding away with set after set after set, they're actually doing much more harm than good.

So what *does* cause optimal muscle growth, then? The short answer is *overload,* which we'll go over in more detail soon.

MYTH & MISTAKE #5:
WASTING TIME WITH THE WRONG EXERCISES

In case you didn't know, most of what your gym has to offer in terms of workout machines and contraptions is worthless. Why? Because they just don't stimulate the muscles like free weights do. (*Free weights,* by the way, are objects like dumbbells, barbells, adjustable pulleys, and lat pull-down setups that can be moved in three-dimensional space.)

There's something oddly effective about the body having to freely manipulate weight, unaided, against the pull of gravity. Nobody ever built a great chest by just pounding away on the Pec Deck and Machine Press—they used barbells and dumbbells.

More specifically, the most effective muscle-building exercises are known as *compound exercises*. They're called compound exercises because they involve multiple muscle groups. Examples of compound exercises are the Squat, Deadlift, and Bench Press. The opposite of a compound exercise is an *isolation exercise*, which involves one muscle group only. Examples of isolation exercises are the Cable Fly, Tricep Kickback, and Leg Extension.

Numerous scientific studies have confirmed the benefits of compound exercises over isolation exercises. One such study was conducted at Ball State University in 2000[3], and it went like this:

Two groups of men trained with weights for ten weeks. Group one did four compound upper-body exercises, while group two did the same plus bicep curls and tricep extensions (isolation exercises).

After the training period, both groups increased strength and size, but which do you think had bigger arms? The answer is neither. The additional isolation training performed by group two produced no additional effect on arm strength or circumference. The takeaway is that by overloading your entire system, you cause everything to grow.

Charles Poliquin, trainer to world-class athletes like Olympians and professional sports players, is fond of saying that in order to gain an inch on your arm, you have to gain ten pounds of muscle. His point is the most effective way to build a muscular, strong body is with *systemic* overload, not localized training.

Now, I'm not saying that bicep curls and tricep extensions are bad. I do both. But if your weight training program isn't built around compound training, you're only making a fraction of the gains possible.

People that make the mistake of doing exercises that produce less-than-optimum gains often fall victim to a similarly counter-productive myth: that you have to constantly change up your routine to make gains. This is complete nonsense peddled by the garbage workout mags. You're in the gym to improve your muscle tone and get stronger, and that requires three simple things: lift progressively heavier weights, eat correctly, and give your body sufficient rest.

Regularly changing exercises simply isn't necessary because your goals limit the exercises that you should be doing. If you're new to weightlifting and want to build a solid foundation, you will be doing the same exercises every week, and they will include things like Squats, Deadlifts, Bench Presses, Dumbbell Presses, Barbell Curls, and others. If you're lifting correctly, your strength will skyrocket, and you will steadily gain lean, sexy muscle…so why would you change your routine?

MYTH & MISTAKE #6:
TRAINING LIKE AN IDIOT

One of the most painful sights in gyms is the hordes of ego lifters spastically throwing around weights with reckless abandon. I cringe not only out of pity but out of the anticipation of injuries that could strike at any moment.

While it might seem like another shocking generality, it's true nonetheless: Most people don't have a clue as to the proper form of exercises. And, this lack of knowledge stunts their gains; causes unnecessary wear and tear on ligaments, tendons, and joints; and opens the door to debilitating injuries (especially as weights get heavy on things like the shoulders, elbows, knees, and back).

Some of these people just don't know any better, and some are more interested in looking cool than in making real gains. That's fine. As a part of *Thinner Leaner Stronger*, you're going to watch videos that show you exactly how to do each exercise to ensure maximum muscle stimulation and safety.

MYTH & MISTAKE #7:
TRAINING LIKE A WUSSY

Building a great body is a pain in the butt. It takes considerable time, effort, discipline, and dedication. I don't care what anybody tells you—it doesn't come easy.

Quite frankly, most people train like wussies. They don't want to push themselves. They don't want to exert too much effort. And of course, they make no gains. They come in each day an exact duplicate of the last. Eventually, they quit out of despair and frustration.

Well, they are giving in to one of our most primal instincts: We humans instinctively avoid pain and discomfort and seek pleasure and ease in life. But, if we let that inclination color our workouts, we're doomed.

Working out correctly is a bit counter-intuitive. It's intense and uncomfortable. Sometimes you just don't want to do that final exercise. Sometimes you dread that next set of squats. Muscle soreness can be annoying. Sometimes joints and tendons can ache.

But, these things are all just a part of the game, and if you push through them and resolve that your body IS going to meet the goals you set for it, then you're going to make great gains—period.

MYTH & MISTAKE #8:
EATING TO STAY WEAK OR GET FAT

As you've probably heard, your body changes *outside* of the gym, and that requires sufficient rest and nutrition.

What most people don't know, however, is what constitutes sufficient nutrition. Most people are way, way off. They don't eat enough calories (or eat way too many), they don't get enough protein (or way too much), they eat unhealthy carbs and fats, and they don't schedule and proportion their meals correctly.

If you don't eat enough calories and get enough protein, carbs, and fats throughout the day, your muscles *simply don't grow bigger or stronger*. It doesn't matter how hard you train; if you don't eat enough, you won't gain any muscle to speak of.

On the other hand, if you eat too many calories, eat unhealthy carbs and fats, and don't know how to proportion and plan your meals properly, you can gain muscle, but it will be hidden underneath an ugly sheath of unnecessary fat.

When you know how to eat properly, you make eye-popping gains in muscle growth while staying lean, and you can lose layers of fat while maintaining, if not, increasing muscle mass.

THE BOTTOM LINE

Well, you've just learned the path to fitness misery: Grind away for hours in the gym, do tons of sets, do the wrong exercises with bad form, don't push yourself too hard, and eat incorrectly.

These myths and mistakes are responsible for untold frustration, discouragement, confusion, and lack of results. Over the years, it's surprising how many people I've seen quit due to making one or more of these mistakes.

So, if that's how to do it wrong, how do you correctly go about building muscle? Continue to find out.

6

THE REAL SCIENCE OF MUSCLE GROWTH

THE LAWS OF MUSCLE GROWTH are as certain, observable, and irrefutable as those of physics.

When you throw a ball in the air, it comes down. When you take the correct actions inside and outside the gym, your muscles grow. It's really that simple, and these laws apply regardless of how much you might think your genetics are against you.

These principles have been known and followed for decades by people who built some of the greatest physiques we've ever seen. Some of these laws will be in direct contradiction of things you've read or heard, but fortunately, they require no leaps of faith or reflection. They are *practical*. Follow them, and you get immediate results. Once these rules have worked for you, you will know they're true.

THE FIRST LAW OF MUSCLE GROWTH:
MUSCLES GROW *ONLY* IF THEY'RE *FORCED* TO

This law may seem obvious and not worth stating, but trust me, most people just don't get it. By lifting weights, you are actually causing tiny tears (known as "micro-tears") in the muscle fibers, which the body then repairs, adapting the muscles to better handle the stimulus that caused the damage. This is the process by which muscles grow (scientifically termed *hypertrophy*).

If a workout causes too few micro-tears in the fibers, then little muscle growth will occur as a result because the body figures it doesn't need to grow to deal again with such a minor stimulus. If a workout causes too many micro-tears, then the body will fail to fully repair the muscles, and muscle growth will be stunted. If a workout causes optimal micro-tearing but the body isn't supplied with sufficient nutrition or rest, little muscle growth will occur.

For optimal muscle growth, you must train in such a way that causes optimal micro-tearing and then you must feed your body what it needs to grow and give it the proper amount of rest.

THE SECOND LAW OF MUSCLE GROWTH: MUSCLES GROW FROM OVERLOAD, NOT FATIGUE OR "PUMP"

While many people think a burning sensation in their muscles is indicative of an intense, "growth-inducing" workout, it's actually *not* an indicator of an optimum workout.

The "burn" you feel is simply an infusion of lactic acid in the muscle, which is produced as a muscle burns its energy stores.

Muscle pump is also not a good indicator of future muscle growth. The pump you feel when training is a result of blood being "trapped" in the muscles, and while it's a good psychological boost and studies have shown that it can help with protein synthesis (the process by which cells build proteins), it's not a primary driver of growth.

What triggers muscle growth, then? Overload. Muscles must be given a clear reason to grow, and overload is the best reason. This makes sense logically, but is also supported by science. In a meta-analysis of 140 related studies, Arizona State University found that a progression in resistance optimizes strength gains and muscle growth. Researchers also found that working in the 4-6 rep range (80% of 1RM) is most effective for those that train regularly[4].

Therefore, building muscle and getting stronger requires lifting heavy weights, and doing short, intense sets of relatively low reps. This type of training causes optimal micro-tearing for strength and growth gains, and forces the body to adapt.

Now, if the idea of lifting "heavy" weights scares you, I understand. Most women are accustomed to using the Barbie dumbbells, but therein lies a big problem and Big Lie of women's fitness. By training with very light weights, you simply can't cause enough damage to your muscle fibers to result in muscle growth, which means your muscles just don't change. You don't get stronger, and your muscles don't grow, and thus you don't SEE any difference—no improved "tone" or "shape."

Doing a bunch of back-to-back, light-weight sets is for the magazine-reading crowd. Such training techniques are often done with isolation exercises, further limiting their effectiveness. They simply do NOT stimulate growth like simple, heavy sets do. And that's the only reason we're in the gym, right?

The same goes for the confused crowd of "muscle confusion" advocates who say you need to change your routine every week or two. This is pure nonsense. As you'll soon learn, you can make incredible gains by doing the same proven, exercises every week, steadily increasing weight and reps (overload).

THE THIRD LAW OF MUSCLE GROWTH:
MUSCLES GROW *OUTSIDE* THE GYM

Most training programs have you training way too often. They play into the common misconception that building muscle is simply a matter of lifting excessively. People who have fallen into this bad habit need to realize that if they did *less* of the *right thing*, they would get *more* of a *good thing*. Yes, I said that right: Do less to get more.

How does that work? Well, muscles grow during the recovery period—the period of time between workouts of the same muscle groups. When you overload your muscles, your body gets to work adapting them to overcome future overloads, and to do the job correctly, it needs sufficient rest and nutrition.

If you wait too few days before training a muscle group again, you can actually lose strength and muscle size. If you allow your muscles enough recuperation time (and eat correctly), however, you will experience maximum strength and size gains.

The amount of sleep that you get also plays a crucial role in gaining muscle. While your body produces growth hormone on a 24-hour cycle, much of it is produced during sleep, and this is a major driver of muscle growth.

Good general advice is to get enough sleep each night that you wake up feeling rested and aren't tired throughout the day. For most people, this means 6-12 hours of sleep each night.

THE FOURTH LAW OF MUSCLE GROWTH:
MUSCLES GROW ONLY IF THEY'RE PROPERLY FED

How important is nutrition? Nutrition is nearly *everything*. Simply put, your diet determines about 70-80% of how you look (muscular or scrawny, lean or flabby). You could do the perfect workouts and give your muscles the perfect amount of rest time, but if you don't eat correctly, *your muscles won't grow bigger or stronger—period*.

Almost everyone gets this wrong. They just don't give their body what it needs to rapidly build muscle. Sure, we all know to eat protein, but how much? How many times per day? Which kinds? What about carbs—which kinds are best? How much? When should they be eaten to maximize gains? And fats…are they important? How much do you need, and what are the best ways to get them? Last but not least, how many calories should you be eating every day? How large should your meals be as the day goes on?

Thinner Leaner Stronger is going to give you the definitive answers to all of these questions and more, so that you never make a diet mistake again.

THE BOTTOM LINE

Building lean muscle is, in essence, just a matter of following these four laws religiously: lift hard, lift heavy, get sufficient rest, and feed your body correctly. That's how you build a strong, healthy, lean body. As you see, it's much simpler than the marketing departments of supplement companies and their magazines want you to think.

The workouts you will be doing as a part of *Thinner Leaner Stronger* are built on these four principles, and if you set aside any doubts or other ideas that you may have and give these methods an honest try, you'll be amazed at how quickly your body will change.

7

THE 5 BIGGEST FAT LOSS MYTHS & MISTAKES

FOR THOUSANDS OF YEARS NOW, a lean, toned body has been the holy grail of the female physique. It was a hallmark of the ancient heroes and goddesses, and it has remained a revered quality, idolized in pop culture, achieved by few, but coveted by many.

With obesity rates over 36% here in America (and steadily rising), it would appear that getting lean and becoming one of the "physically elite" must require a level of knowledge, discipline, and sacrifice beyond what most humans are capable of.

Well, this simply isn't true. The knowledge is easy enough to understand (in fact, you're learning everything you need to know in this book). Sure, it requires discipline and some "sacrifice" in that no, you can't eat three pizzas a week and have a flat, tight stomach, but here's the kicker: When you're training and dieting correctly, you will *enjoy* the lifestyle. You will look forward to the gym each day. You won't mind the weeks of dieting to lose weight. You won't feel compelled to eat a bunch of junk food or desserts (even though you will be able to have them).

Simply put: You will look and feel better than you ever have before—and this will continue to improve every month—and you will find it infinitely more pleasurable and valuable than being lazy and addicted to ice cream and potato chips. When you can get into this "zone," you can do whatever you want with your body—the results are inevitable; it's just a matter of time.

But, most people never find this sweet spot. Why? Well, the most practical answer to that question is twofold: 1) They don't have a strong enough desire to get there (they don't have their "inner game" sorted out), and 2) they lack the know-how required to make it happen, which leads to poor results, which kills discipline and makes sacrifices no longer worthwhile.

In this chapter, I want to address the five most common myths and mistakes of burning fat. Like those of building muscle, these fallacies and errors have snuck into our heads via magazines, advertising, trainers, friends, etc. Let's dispel them once and for all so that they can't block your path to having the toned body that you desire.

MYTH & MISTAKE #1:
COUNTING CALORIES IS UNNECESSARY

I don't know how many people I've consulted who wanted to lose weight but didn't want to have to count calories. This statement is about as logical as saying that you want to drive across the country but don't want to have to pay attention to your gas tank.

Now, I won't be too hard on them because they didn't even know what a calorie was, and they just didn't want to be bothered with having to count anything. Well, whether you want to call it "counting" calories or whatever else, in order to lose weight, you have to regulate food intake.

In order to lose fat, you must keep your body burning more energy than you're feeding it, and the energy potential of food is measured in calories. Eat too many calories—give your body more potential energy than it needs—and it has no incentive to burn fat.

What people are actually objecting to with counting calories is trying to figure out what to eat while on the run every day or what to buy when rushing through the grocery store. When they have a 30-minute window for lunch and run to the nearest restaurant, they don't want to have to analyze the menu to figure out calories. They just order something that sounds healthy and hope for the best. But, little do they know that their "quick, healthy" meal has hundreds of more calories than they should've eaten. Repeat that for dinner, and a day of weight loss progress is totally lost.

Well, that's the problem—not "having to count calories." People make it unnecessarily hard by failing to plan out and prepare meals. It might seem easier to just heat up some leftovers for lunch and carry on with the day, but that convenience comes with a price: little or no weight loss.

MYTH & MISTAKE #2:
DO CARDIO = LOSE WEIGHT

Every day I see overweight people grinding away on the cardio machines. And, week after week goes by with them looking the same.

They are under the false impression that idly going through the motions on an elliptical machine or stationary bike will somehow flip a magical fat loss switch in the body. Well, that's not how it works.

You already know how to lose fat (make your body burn more energy than it gets from food), and cardio can *enhance* fat loss in two ways: 1) by burning calories and 2) by speeding up your metabolic rate.

To clarify point #2, your body burns a certain number of calories regardless of any physical activity, and this is called your *basal metabolic rate.* Your total caloric expenditure for a day would be your BMR plus the energy expended during any physical activities.

When your metabolism is said to "speed up" or "slow down," what this means is that your basal metabolic rate has gone up or down. That is, your body is burning more calories while at rest (allowing you to eat more calories without putting on fat) or burning less (making it easier to eat too much and gain fat).

But here's the thing with cardio: If you don't eat correctly, that nightly run or bike ride won't necessarily save you.

Let's say you're trying to lose weight and are unwittingly eating six hundred calories more than your body burns during the day. You go jogging for thirty minutes at night, which burns about three hundred calories. That leaves you with a daily excess of three hundred calories, and the small jump in your metabolic rate from the cardio won't be enough to burn that up plus burn fat stores.

You could continue like this for *years* and never get lean. As a matter of fact, you'll probably slowly put on weight instead.

MYTH & MISTAKE #3:
CHASING THE FADS

The Atkins Diet. The South Beach Diet. The Paleo Diet. The HCG Diet (this one really makes me cringe). The Hollywood Diet. The Body Type Diet. It seems like a new one pops up every month or two. I can't keep up these days.

While not all "latest and greatest" diets are bad (Paleo is quite healthy, actually), the sheer abundance of fad diets being touted by fit actors is making people pretty confused as to what the "right way" to lose weight is (and understandably so).

The result is that many people jump from diet to diet, failing to get the results they desire. And, they buy into some pretty stupid stuff simply because they don't understand the physiology of metabolism and fat loss. The rules are the rules, and no fancy names or snake oil supplements will help you get around them.

In this book, you're going to learn how simple getting lean really is. Once you understand the basic principles of why the body stores fat and how to coax it into shedding it, you'll see how asinine many of the fad diets taking gyms by storm really are.

MYTH & MISTAKE #4:

DOING LOW WEIGHT AND HIGH REPS BUILDS "LEAN MUSCLE"

This myth goes like this: If you want that lean, toned look, you want to do a BUNCH of reps with low weight. This is just plain wrong.

To be honest, I can't think of a reason why anyone would want to do a routine based on low weight and high reps. While there's a never-ending debate as to what rep ranges are best for hypertrophy (muscle growth), research has shown that doing more than fifteen reps causes little to no improvement in muscle power or size due to insufficient overload[5]. It only improves muscle endurance (the ability to contract over and over).

Being lean is a matter of having low body fat. Nothing else. Building muscle is a matter of overloading the muscles and letting them repair. Combine the two and voila, you look extremely "toned."

Light weights don't overload the muscles no matter how many reps you do (remember that *fatigue* doesn't trigger growth). No overload = no growth.

Heavy weights, however, *do* overload the muscles and force them to adapt. Optimum overload and proper nutrition and rest = fast, noticeable muscle growth.

So, even if you don't want to gain too much muscle, the fastest route to that goal is *heavy weight*. Once you're there, you can simply maintain what you have (more on that later).

How heavy should you be going, though? How many exercises, sets, and reps should you do? You'll find out soon!

MYTH & MISTAKE #5:

SPOT REDUCTION

How many people have you seen doing crunches "to get a six pack"? How many woman try to target their butts and thighs to "burn away the fat"?

Well, that's not how it works. You can't reduce fat in any particular area of your body by targeting it with exercises. You can reduce fat by proper dieting, and your body will decide how it comes off (which areas will become lean first and which will be stubborn). Our bodies are all genetically programmed differently, and there's nothing we can do to change that.

We all have our "fat spots" that annoy us to no end, and that's just genetics for you. Some guys I know store every last pound in their hips while others are fortunate to have their fat accumulate more in their chest, shoulders, and arms more so than over their stomachs.

Rest assured, however, that you *can* lose as much fat all over your body as you want, and you *can* get as toned as you want; you'll just have to be patient and let your body lean out in the way it is programmed to.

THE BOTTOM LINE

Like building muscle, many people approach fat loss completely wrong and thus fail to achieve their weight goals. But, just like building muscle, the laws of fat loss are actually very simple and incredibly effective. Carry on to learn the laws and how to put them to work for you.

8

THE REAL SCIENCE OF HEALTHY FAT LOSS

BEFORE GETTING INTO THE LAWS of fat loss, I want to share some insight into how your body views fat versus muscle. Your body views fat as an asset and muscle as a liability. Why?

Because evolution has taught the body that having fat means being able to survive the times when food is scarce. Many thousands of years ago, when our ancestors were roaming the wilderness, they sometimes journeyed for days without food, and their bodies lived off fat stores. Starving, they would finally kill an animal and feast, and their bodies knew to prepare for the next bout of starvation by storing fat. Having fat was literally a matter of life and death.

This genetic programming is still in us, ready to be used. If you starve your body, it will burn fat to stay alive, but it will also slow down its metabolic rate to conserve energy, becoming fully prepared to store fat once you start feeding it higher quantities of food again.

Muscle, on the other hand, is viewed as a liability because it costs energy to maintain. While there is much debate as to the exact numbers in terms of calories, your body burns more energy due to a pound of muscle than a pound of fat. Thus, your body doesn't want to carry more muscle than it has to because it knows that it has to keep it properly fed, and this requires calories that it may or may not get.

So, what does this mean for fat loss? Well, it means that you have to show your body that it has no reason to store excess fat and, in a sense, coax it to the level that you desire. The same goes for building muscle: If you don't provide your body with the perfect building conditions (proper training, proper nutrition, and proper rest), it will be inclined to simply not grow its muscles.

All right, let's dive into the fundamental laws of fat loss.

THE FIRST LAW OF FAT LOSS: EAT LESS THAN YOU EXPEND = LOSE WEIGHT

Fat loss is just a science of numbers, much like gaining muscle.

No matter what anyone tells you, getting toned boils down to nothing more than manipulating a simple mathematical formula: energy consumed versus energy expended. As you would expect, this has been determined beyond the shadow of a doubt by many studies, including the definitive study conducted by the University of Lausanne[6].

When you give your body more calories (potential energy) than it burns off, it stores fat. When you give your body less calories than it burns throughout the day, it must make up for that deficit by burning its own energy stores (fat), leading to the ultimate goal, fat loss. It doesn't even matter what you eat—if your calories are right, you'll lose weight. Don't believe me?

Professor Mark Haub, from Kansas State University, conducted a weight loss study on himself in 2010. He started the study at 211 pounds and 33.4% body fat (overweight). He calculated that he would need to eat about 1,800 calories per day to lose weigh without starving himself. He followed this protocol for two months and lost 27 pounds, but here's the kicker: while he had one protein shake and a couple servings of vegetables each day, two-thirds of his daily calories came from Twinkies, Little Debbies, Doritos, sugary cereals, and Oreos—a "convenience store diet," as he called it. And he not only lost the weight, but his "bad" cholesterol, or LDL, dropped 20 percent and his "good" cholesterol, or HDL, increased 20 percent.

Now, Haub doesn't recommend this diet, of course, but he was doing it to prove a point. When it comes to fat loss, calories are king.

Healthy fat loss *isn't* as simple as drastically cutting calories, however. If you eat too little, your body will go into "starvation mode" and sure, it will lose fat, but you will also lose muscle. Plus, worst of all, your metabolic rate will slow down, and once you start eating more, you'll quickly gain the fat back (and sometimes even more than you lost). This is what leads to yo-yo dieting.

So yes, you will need to watch your calories. Yes, you will get used to feeling a little hungry (at least for the first week or two of dieting to lose weight). Yes, you will have to stay disciplined and skip the daily desserts.

But, if you do it right, you can get super lean without losing muscle...or even while gaining muscle (yes, this can be done—more on that later).

THE SECOND LAW OF FAT LOSS: EAT ON A SCHEDULE THAT WORKS BEST FOR YOU

This law might come as a bit of a surprise to you.

Most meal scheduling advice goes like this: to lose weight, you have to eat multiple small meals per day.

The reason often given is that eating like this will speed up your metabolism and thus your weight loss.

It seems to make sense on the surface—by putting food in our bodies every few hours, it has to constantly work to break it down, which should speed up our metabolism, right?

Well, not really.

In an extensive review of literature, researchers looked at scores of studies comparing the metabolic effects of a wide variety of eating patterns, ranging from 1-17 meals per day[7]. In terms of 24-hour energy expenditure, they found no difference between nibbling and gorging. Small meals caused small, short metabolic boosts, and large meals caused larger, longer boosts, and by the end of each day, they balanced out in terms of total calories burned.

We can also look to a study conducted by the University of Ontario, which split into two dietary groups: 3 meals per day and 3 meals plus 3 snacks per day, with both in a caloric restriction for weight loss[8]. After 8 weeks, 16 participants completed the study and researchers found no significant difference in average weight loss, fat loss, and muscle loss.

As you know, the bottom line is fat loss is how much you eat. When you eat it has little bearing on the equation.

So, the most important aspect of meal scheduling is that you work out what makes dieting most enjoyable for you, and what fits your lifestyle. This way you can actually stick to your diet, which is what matters in the end.

That said, if you can, I actually recommend that you break up your daily caloric needs into 4-6 meals. Why?

Because my experience coaching hundreds of people has taught me that those that ate only 2-3 meals per day found it very hard to control their calories due to hunger, which led to overeating. By eating 4-6 meals per day, however, people found it much easier to stick to their diet plans because they never felt famished.

I also prefer more, smaller meals, simply because I don't like the feeling of having to stuff myself full of feed to meet my nutritional needs.

If you would rather eat fewer, larger meals every day, however, feel free to do that. Except for your pre- and post-workout nutrition (you'll learn more about this soon), meal timing is completely negotiable. If you're new to this game, then I recommend you simply start with eating 4-6 meals per day.

THE THIRD LAW OF FAT LOSS: USE CARDIO TO HELP BURN FAT

As you know, doing cardio doesn't equal burning fat. It can accelerate fat loss by burning calories and by speeding up your metabolic rate, but whether you actually lose fat or not will be determined by your daily caloric intake and expenditure.

Now, with that being said, most women find cardio necessary in order to get into the "super lean" category (15% body fat and under) because you can only cut your calories so much before you start to lose strength and muscle and feel exhausted. Some people, however, don't need to bother much with cardio—they simply regulate their calories and get as lean as they want. This is really just a matter of genetics and individual physiology.

THE BOTTOM LINE

Believe it or not, fat loss depends on these three laws and no others. The U.S. weight loss market generates over *$60 billion per year*, and, drugs and invasive surgeries aside, any and all workable weight loss methods rely on the three simple rules you just read to achieve results.

Sure, you can get fancy and count "points" instead of calories, can come up with all kinds of creative recipes, can have your miniature desserts, and so on. Regardless, the fundamentals of fat loss don't need a fancy name or marketing campaign. They really are this simple.

9

THE INNER AND
OUTER GAMES OF
HEALTH AND FITNESS

THERE'S SOMETHING MYSTICAL ABOUT THREE months of training.

That's when many people quit. Yup, strangely enough, I've seen dozens of people over the years make it to three or four months and, for one reason or another, just disappear. Some people got sick and never returned. Others decided to take a week off and turned it into a permanent break. Others were just plain lazy and started making excuses as to why they didn't really care about being in shape anymore.

Most of these people had one thing in common: They weren't happy with their gains, and without visible results for their efforts, it's understandable that their motivation waned. Fortunately for you, you're not going to have this problem. If you follow exactly what you learn in this book, you'll make incredible gains and will feel more motivated after three months than you do right now.

Before we get into the nuts and bolts of training and diet, however, I want you to know that there are two equally important aspects of achieving the body of your dreams, and I call them the "outer game" and "inner game" of training.

The outer game is the physical stuff—how to lift, how to eat, how to rest, and so on—and this is what most trainers, books, and magazines focus on. But the inner game is the less-discussed aspect of training, and if you don't have this squared away, you'll be in for a rough ride.

The inner game is, of course, the mental side of training and diet, and this is what really sets apart the great physiques from the mediocre. Building a killer physique is not a matter of jumping on the bandwagon of some new fad workout program for a few months—it's a matter of adopting a disciplined, orderly approach to how you handle your body, which is quite a lifestyle change for most.

Now, people's biggest mental barriers in this world are *lack of motivation and lack of discipline.* They usually start out full of resolve and intention, but within only a few weeks, their dedication is wavering. That new TV show is starting during gym time... That extra hour of sleep would really hit the spot... A few days off isn't a big deal... Another cheat meal shouldn't hurt too much...

Well, these are the things that lead you down the slippery slope of getting less-than-great results and eventually quitting altogether.

While it's true that some people are just more naturally disciplined than others, anyone can use the simple tricks I'm going to teach you in the next couple of chapters to get mentally prepared to win and to stay the course even when tempted to go astray.

10

HOW TO SET FITNESS GOALS THAT WILL MOTIVATE YOU

THIS IS SO SIMPLE AND clichéd that you'd think it wouldn't need stating, but it does: Before you lift a weight, hop on a treadmill, or cut a calorie, you must have specific, tangible goals set in your mind as to why you're doing it.

People with vague, unrealistic, or uninspiring health or fitness goals (or none at all) are always the first to quit. They're easy to spot, too. They show up randomly and seem to sleepwalk through their training routines, wandering from machine to machine, going through the motions. Week after week, they complain about how hard it is to diet and rant about failing to lose weight.

Let me assure you that anyone who has the type of body that you aspire to has very specific, realistic health and fitness goals and is driven by them, progressing slowly but surely toward them every day. When they meet one goal, they set another goal to stay motivated. This is what we're going to work out for you in this chapter.

People have many different reasons for training. Some like the game of pushing their bodies past its limits. Some want to look good to impress the opposite sex. Some want to feel more confident about themselves. Some want to be healthy and feel good.

The reality is that all of these things are fine reasons to train. Sure, I could give you a nice list of benefits of being in great shape, such as looking great, feeling great, having high energy levels, being highly resistant to sickness and disease, and so on, but the important thing is that you work out very specifically what fires *you* up about training.

We might as well start with what people usually consider more important: the visual. Hey, there's nothing to be ashamed of here. Every single person I know who has built an awesome physique was at least 50% motivated by the looks they wanted.

Sure, having no regard for health and only chasing looks leads to drugs and other undesirable practices, but there's nothing wrong with being motivated by wanting to look a certain way. I value my health highly and am not solely driven by vanity, but I would be lying if I said I don't care as much about the looks. I think being muscular and lean looks awesome, and I feel good when I look in the mirror.

STEP ONE:
WHAT DOES YOUR IDEAL BODY LOOK LIKE?

The first step of establishing your goals is to determine what your ideal body would look like. Not just in your head, but in reality. You need to find pictures of exactly what you want to look like and save them for future reference.

It might seem silly for you to go searching on the internet for pictures of hot woman, but it's important that you have an exact visual image of how you want your body to look. Throwing around words like "lean" and "toned" to describe your goal isn't nearly as motivating as looking at pictures of real bodies that you are working toward.

And here's a fact: If you follow this program exactly and work hard, you can have the type of body you dream of. All it takes is that you dedicate yourself to it and follow the right game plan.

Two good sites to look through for ideal body shots are Simply-Shredded.com (check out the IFBB Bikini Pros) and bodybuilding.com's BodySpace. I'm also building a little collection of my inspiration on Pinterest, which you can find at http://www.pinterest.com/mikebls.

STEP TWO:
WHAT WOULD YOUR IDEAL STATE OF HEALTH BE LIKE?

Now that you've worked out what you want to look like, let's take a look at the other side of this coin: health. Even if looking a certain way is your primary motivation for training, you will soon learn that the health benefits are just as motivating. You're going to feel better physically, you're going to have higher energy levels, you're going to get stronger, you're going to be more mentally alert, you're going to have a stronger sex drive, and more.

Studies such as those conducted by the U.S. National Institute on Aging and the University of Pittsburgh have shown that the stronger your body is, the longer you'll live, and the less likely you are to fall prey to heart disease.

Work out a health goal that you find motivating. Mine is along these lines: *to have a vital, energetic, strong, and disease-free body that lives long and allows me to stay active and enjoy my life to the fullest.* For me, that's what this is all about. I want to live a long life, feel good, watch my future kids grow up, and never suffer from debilitating diseases.

I'm sure your health interests are along the same lines, but feel free to work out your individual goals in whatever words best communicate to you.

STEP THREE:
WHY DO YOU WANT TO ACHIEVE THESE GOALS?

All right, now that you've worked out what you want to look like and what level of health you want, the next question is *why*. What are the reasons for achieving those goals? This is completely personal, so write whatever is most motivating to you.

Maybe you want to boost your confidence; maybe you want to better enjoy sports you play or physically taxing hobbies of yours; maybe you want to get more attention from the opposite sex; maybe you want to feel the satisfaction of overcoming physical barriers; maybe you want to be able to participate in physical activities with your kids; hell, maybe you want to just be able to do a few pull-ups. Whatever your reasons, just write them all down.

For the sake of simplicity, first write the "whys" for the looks goals, then focus on the health goal.

THE BOTTOM LINE

By doing these three simple steps, you'll have created a powerful "motivation sheet" that will always point the way. When you feel a bit tired and are dreading the gym, you can just look at that sheet, and you'll probably change your mind. When you're out with friends, watching them stuff themselves silly while you're eating your fish and vegetables, you'll know exactly why you're doing it.

This is the simple yet powerful formula that I've used to keep myself continually motivated to train and diet for nearly a decade now. Over the years, my goals have changed, but I've always ensured that I knew where I was going and why. Chances are you will greatly benefit by doing the same.

11

THE CODE OF A GOOD TRAINING PARTNER

WORKING OUT WITH A BAD partner sucks. A lot.

Working out with a good partner is great, however, and it's actually a very important aspect of staying motivated and on track. Not only does having a partner hold you accountable to show up (if you skip, you're not only letting yourself down but your partner too), but it also helps to have someone to spot you on certain exercises, to push you for another rep, or to go up in weight.

A good partner can make a big difference as time goes on. Those days that you would've skipped solo but went because of your partner will add up to real gains, as will the times where you wouldn't have gone up in weight or wouldn't have pushed yourself for those last couple of reps.

So, I *highly* recommend that you find someone to work out with before you start, and the two of you should agree to the following code.

THE CODE OF A GOOD TRAINING PARTNER

1. I will show up on time for every workout, and if I can't avoid missing one, I'll let my partner know as soon as I know.

2. I will come to the gym to *train*—not to chat. When we're in the gym, we focus on our workouts, we're always ready to spot each other, and we get our work done efficiently.

3. I will train hard to set a good example for my partner.

4. I will push my partner to do more than she thinks she can. It's my job to motivate her to do more weight and more reps than she believes possible.

5. I will be supportive of my partner and will compliment her on her gains.

6. I won't let my partner get out of a workout easily. I will reject any excuses that are short of an actual emergency or commitment that can't be rescheduled, and I will insist that she comes and trains. In the case where there's a valid excuse, I'll offer to train at a different time so we can get our workout in (if at all possible).

Such a code might seem silly, but if you and your partner keep to these six points, you'll be doing each other a huge favor and will make great gains together.

On the flip side, if your partner can't keep to these points—if she's inconsistent in showing up, if she's more interested in chatting than training, if she trains lethargically, if she doesn't push you to do more, etc.—then she's a *bad training partner* and is actually doing more harm to you than good. You need to get her onto this program and follow the above code, or you need to find someone else to train with who embodies the above commitments.

12

IF YOU CAN'T
MEASURE IT, YOU
DON'T KNOW IT

SIR WILLIAM THOMSON, ALSO KNOWN as Lord Kelvin, was an ingenious physicist and engineer, and he said that when you can measure something and express it in numbers, you know something about it; but when you can't measure it or express it numbers, your knowledge is lacking.

This insight is actually very applicable to training and dieting. If you can measure your progress (or lack thereof) and express it in real numbers, then you know if you're going in the right direction or not. If you don't have any way to measure progress, then you're going at it blind, hoping for the best.

One of the most effective protections against getting stuck in a rut of no gains is keeping a training and diet journal. I know this may sound a bit overboard at first, but trust me, it makes a *huge* difference. I consider it absolutely *vital* to making long-term gains.

Let me ask you a question. What is the most frustrating thing women run into with their training and dieting? Hands down, the answer to that question is *hitting a plateau and getting stuck in a rut.* Nothing is more annoying than taking the time and effort to hit the gym every day just to look the same week after week.

And what about dieting? What's the most frustrating thing women run into here? *Not losing weight or building muscle as quickly as they should be.* Many women think they're eating right but that for some "inexplicable" reason, they aren't losing much fat or gaining much muscle.

Well, let me warn you that if you don't keep a training and diet journal, you're almost *guaranteed* to run into these problems. You're going to plateau in your training, and you're going to forever struggle with eating correctly (especially losing weight). Why?

THE TRAINING JOURNAL

Building your ideal body takes time. As the old adage goes, it's a marathon, not a sprint. Now, if you know what you're doing, you can make incredible gains and enjoy the ride, but no matter how you look at it, it takes a real investment of time and effort.

The key to growing your muscles is to *always get stronger*. For your muscles to get stronger and adapt to progressively heavier weights, they must grow—it's that simple. Now, the tricky thing about muscle strength is that it comes slowly, bit by bit. If you're just starting out, you're going to see huge jumps in strength for the first several months, but eventually your strength gains will slow down. From that point on, you will have to consciously work for every pound of improvement on your lifts. And, of course, this is where things get hazy for people who don't keep journals, and they end up falling into the routine of the same exercises, same weights, and same reps every week. Well this is a great way to make no gains, along with doing different excercises every week with random weights, which doesn't allow for any measure¬ment of progress whatsoever.

How do you avoid this? That's where your journal comes in. Your goal each week is to do just a little more than last week. That doesn't necessarily mean more weight, because going up in weight on every exercise every week would be impossible. It also means reps. More reps eventually turns into more weight. For example, if you squatted 90 pounds for 8 reps on week 1, for 9 reps on week 2, and for 10 reps on week 3, you should be able to come in on week 4 and do 8 reps of 100-105 pounds. The process then restarts, and you move on up to 110 pounds, 115, and so on. This is how strength is built—one rep at a time.

If you don't keep a journal, however, you probably won't know what you did the week before. Sure, you might make a mental note of the certain exercises, but what about everything else? You need to approach *all* exercises in the same way. Your mantra should be, "One more rep!" If you can get *one* more rep on an exercise than you did last week (while maintaining proper form), pat yourself on the back, because you've made progress. If you can't do any more than the week before, don't despair, but you need to push harder the next week. If you're stuck for several weeks, you need to check your nutrition and rest, because something is off.

HOW TO KEEP A TRAINING JOURNAL

So how do you keep a training journal? Simple. You can download an application for your iPod or phone (I like *Gym Buddy* or *JEFit*), or you can keep it old school and get a notebook.

In the notebook, write a series of things for each training day: how many weeks it's been since you took a week off to rest and the day, date, and body part(s) you're going to be training that day. You should also weigh yourself once or twice a week (in the morning, in the nude, after the bathroom, and on an empty stomach) and record it in your book.

You then list out the exercises you're going to do and look at the previous week. You assess whether you're going up in reps or weight this week (you'll learn more about this soon) and then start your first exercise, writing down what you did. You move through your workout this way, always looking back to ensure that you are striving to do more reps or more weight than the week before. Here's an example of how I kept my written journal before switching to an app:

Week 4

192 lbs

8/14/11

Monday

Chest

Bench Press – 275 x 4, x 4, x 4 (feel strong)

Incline Dumbbell Press – 110 x 5, x 5, x 4

Flat Dumbbell Press – 110 x 5, x 5, x5

Pretty simple, right? I sometimes make notes if I felt particularly strong or weak on an exercise, if I struggled heavily with a set, if some kind of ache or pain was bothering me, if I didn't sleep well the night before, etc.

Keeping your journal like this allows you to always have your eye on improvement and to never fall backward or get stuck (and if this does happen, you can discover very specific reasons why and find remedies that will help you bust out of a rut).

There's really nothing else to the training journal. Good apps allow you to track all the same things and also give you nifty graphs to show your progress.

THE DIET JOURNAL

As you'll soon learn, dieting is a very precise activity, especially when you're trying to lose weight. It requires that you split an exact daily requirement of calories, protein, carbs, and fats into several meals each day, with certain meals meeting specific nutritional criteria.

The easiest way to do this is to eat the same food every meal, every day. While this may sound really boring, it has its benefits: It's easy to prepare for, easy to follow, and doesn't require any "on the spot" calorie counting, tracking, or adjusting. If you don't mind doing it, it'll make your life WAY easier. Some people find this agonizingly boring, however; they need some variety in their diets, which is fine, but the variety must be *planned*, not spontaneous.

As you can imagine, trying to figure out calories, protein, carbs, and fats on the fly, in the hustle and bustle of work and everything else, is almost impossible. How many calories are actually in that chicken salad you just ordered at the restaurant that your friends wanted to go to? (More than you probably think.) What about the handful of chips you just ate as an "unscheduled" snack? And the Starbucks latte? The little bag of pretzels? This is how dieting to lose weight utterly fails...one unplanned calorie at a time.

So, how can you have some variety and still follow your diet precisely and thus lose weight (or build muscle while staying lean)? That's what the diet journal is for. The primary use of the diet journal isn't to just *record* what you've eaten throughout the day, but to *plan* out your meals for each day (and then record what you actually end up eating, of course).

Once you know how many calories and how much protein, carbs, and fats you should be eating each day, you can plan out your meals using a nutrition facts database online, such as www.calorieking.com and caloriecount.about.com (my two favorites).

I like to come up with a few different breakfast, lunch, and dinner options and then rotate them throughout the week. You can then shop for and prepare them as needed. I recommend doing this once or twice per week, planning and preparing a week's worth of meals in one or two days per week (I like Sundays and Wednesdays).

Now, for the actual journal itself, there are many phone, tablet, and Web apps out there built for this, but I like to just use Word (or you can use Google's free version, found in their Google Drive app—love this app!). I've also used plain old notebooks.

In your journal, write out the following for each day:

1. Your dietary target for calories, protein, carbs, and fats.

2. The foods you plan on eating for each meal with the total calories, protein, carbs, and fats noted.

3. A note if you stuck to the planned meal or not. You can simply put a check mark next to the meal that you planned if you stuck to it, but if you had to deviate (which you want to avoid, but sometimes can't help), you should note what you ate instead along with the calories, protein, carbs, and fats.

This would look something like this:

10/3/2011

Monday

Targets:

1,600 calories

180 grams of protein

150 grams of carbs

30 grams of fat

Meals:

✓ 7AM–Meal #1:

(Pre-workout meal)

1 cup of rice milk

30g whey protein

30g protein

25g carbs

6g fat

270 calories

✓ <u>9AM–Meal #2:</u>

(Post-workout smoothie)

1 cup of rice milk

1 banana

1 scoop of protein powder

30g protein

50 carbs

2.5g fat

342 calories

(And so on throughout the day, breaking down each meal.)

As the old proverb goes, "If you fail to plan, you plan to fail." This is very true with diet. It is basically impossible to get lean and strong without planning and preparing in the way I've just described, and this is why most people fail to achieve the results they desire.

13

INTENSITY AND FOCUS— YOUR TWO SECRET WEAPONS

IF YOU'VE TRAINED BEFORE, YOU know what makes a great workout: pushing yourself to the limit with the weights feeling light. Nothing distracts you, and you are fully in the moment, enjoying the blood engorging your muscles. You feel strong and tight.

The secret to having this kind of workout every day is lifting with *intensity* and *focus*. Training with maximum intensity and focus will enable you to lift the heaviest weights possible and thus literally force your muscles to grow.

What do I mean by intensity and focus, though? Does it mean grunting loudly with each rep with heavy metal blaring in your headphones? While some who do this actually train pretty intensely, none of the showmanship is necessary.

Intensity is simply the level of physical and mental exertion you give to your workout. It's how intent you are on pushing yourself outside of your comfort zone and making progress. It's your desire to make it through each set no matter what.

A high-intensity workout is one where you feel like you didn't leave anything in the tank. You didn't settle for a lighter weight when you felt you could've gone up. Your mind wasn't wandering elsewhere while you were training. You weren't just robotically going through the motions— you were consciously pushing out every rep and every set. "One more rep!"

By focus, I mean mental concentration, having your mind on your training and not on the TV show you watched last night, the party later that night, the argument with your boyfriend, or whatever else. I don't want to get too "woo-woo" on you and talk about visualizing every lift, but there's definitely something to be said for having one-hundred percent of your attention on moving the weight in front of you. It's "mind over matter," as they say.

The *Thinner Leaner Stronger* training routines are built to help you maintain a high level of intensity and focus. It's much easier to do 8-10 reps at maximum intensity and focus than 20. It's much easier to remain focused and revved up for 45 minutes than 90. But, the routine itself doesn't supply the intensity and focus—you have to.

DON'T GET TOO CHATTY

Training with friends can be great, or it can be a curse. Nothing is worse than training with people who are more interested in hanging out than blasting out a workout.

While there's nothing wrong with talking while resting, don't get carried away in conversation because it'll inevitably be distracting. Your rest times will go too long, and thus your workouts. You'll have your mind on other things when you sit down to do your sets. It's just counterproductive. Save the chatting for after the gym.

14

THE BUILDING BLOCKS OF PROPER NUTRITION

I THINK EVERYONE WHO KNOWS anything about getting lean and strong agrees that nutrition is a massive piece in the puzzle. Some say it's 70% of the game, some say 80% or even 90%. Well, I say it's 100%. Yes, 100%. And training properly, overloading your muscles...that's also 100% of the game. Being properly hydrated is 100%. Having the right attitude is 100% too. (Yeah, we're at 400% so far...)

My point is this: The building blocks of a great body are more like pillars than puzzle pieces. Weaken one enough, and the whole structure collapses. That is, you can't build any appreciable amount of muscle if you don't train correctly. Your muscles won't grow if you don't give your body proper nutritional support. Muscle growth is seriously stunted by dehydration. Your gains will be lackluster if you don't train with the right attitude.

That said, I want you to have an "all or nothing" attitude about achieving your fitness and health goals. I want you to be 100% about each aspect you learn in this program and achieve 100% of the potential results. Let the weak and undisciplined give only 60% in their training, 30% in their dieting, 40% in their attitude. They're going to make you look like a god.

All right, let's now talk about this pillar of achieving your ideal body... *nutrition.*

The nutritional aspect of fitness is incredibly powerful, and it can either work for or against you, multiplying or dividing your end results. It's the series of toll booths along the highway of muscle growth, and if you don't stop and pay each one, you don't get to go any further. It's that simple.

Proper nutrition has nothing to do with loading up on the latest, greatest "advanced muscle building" supplements that clutter the shelves of your local GNC. It's much more than eating a couple good meals per day with some snacks here and there so you don't get hungry. It means following a calculated, regimented eating plan that feeds your body the nutrients it needs to adapt to your training and thus get leaner and stronger.

There are six aspects of nutrition that are of primary concern when trying to build muscle and lose fat. They are calories, protein, carbohydrates, fats, water, and vitamins and minerals. Protein, carbohydrates, and fats are known as "macro-nutrients" (*macro* means "of great size; large"), and how you structure these in your diet is vitally important to your overall results. Of secondary concern to success are vitamins and minerals, which are known as "micro-nutrients," and these are essential for the body's performance of many different physiological processes connected with building muscle and losing fat.

Let's talk more about each of these six aspects of nutrition.

CALORIES

As you already know, a calorie is a measurement of potential energy in a food, whether it comes from protein, carbohydrate, or fat. Like an engine, your body needs fuel to function, and it gets it from food.

A gram of protein is about 4 calories, as is a gram of carbohydrate (regardless of the source, these numbers hold true). A gram of fat is 9 calories. Later in the book you will be creating a diet based on your goals, and you can calculate the calories by multiplying the protein and carbs by 4, and fats by 9.

Your body uses food energy to perform any and all physiological processes that you can imagine. Your brain, lungs, heart, liver, and kidneys require energy to do their jobs. Your muscles require energy to contract and extend. Your body requires energy to build muscle and even to lose fat.

Several factors come into play when determining how much energy your body burns every day (and thus how many calories you should be eating, whether to lose weight, gain muscle, or maintain). Body size, the amount of lean mass, body temperature, the thermic effect of foods (the amount of energy it "costs" to process food for use and storage), stimulants such as caffeine, and your level of physical activity all affect how many calories your body burns every day.

Knowing how to determine your body's caloric needs each day and then how to translate them into specific amounts of protein, carbs, and fats is crucial to maximizing your muscle growth and fat loss. As you can imagine, eating 150 grams of protein per day is much better for achieving muscle growth than eating 65 grams of fat, even though they contain about the same amount of calories.

PROTEIN

Your body needs protein for virtually every "growth" process it engages in. It uses protein to build and repair cells and to produce hormones and enzymes. Your body needs a certain amount of protein to keep its immune system functioning optimally.

Weightlifting places considerable protein demands on the body, and as you gain more lean muscle, your body needs more protein to maintain it. Think of your muscles as protein reservoirs (because that's how your body views them). What do you think happens if you build muscle and then don't provide your body with the protein it needs for its upkeep? That's right—it eats the muscle away and thus reduces its need for protein.

Therefore, eating enough protein every day is rock-bottom fundamental to building muscle and increasing strength. I can't overstate the importance of this, really, because many people just don't get it. They don't pay attention to how much protein they eat each day or miss meals, and figure it's no big deal. Well, it is. In fact, not eating enough protein each day is the easiest way to prevent muscle growth, get stuck in a rut, and quit. I've seen it happen many times.

Protein from meat is also particularly helpful when you're weightlifting. Studies clearly show that meats increase testosterone levels, but scientists aren't sure why. One study had two groups of men, all comparable in health and builds, follow a weightlifting program for twelve weeks. By the end of the program, all had progressed about equally in strength, but only the meat eaters enjoyed significant muscle growth and fat loss.

"Meat" doesn't only mean red meat, by the way. Fish, chicken, turkey, pork, buffalo, and so on all qualify as "meat" in this sense.

I recommend that you stick to the lean varieties of meats as eating a lot of saturated fat just isn't necessary. That means fish, extra-lean cuts of beef (95% lean ground beef, or extra-lean cuts like top sirloin steak, and top and bottom round roast and steak), chicken, turkey, pork tenderloin, and so forth.

If you're vegetarian or vegan, don't worry—the study cited above doesn't mean you're doomed. While you would probably do better if you included meat in your diet, you can still make great gains. I eat quite a bit of vegetarian proteins such as eggs, low-fat cottage cheese (Organic Valley is my favorite), low-fat European style (Greek) yogurt (Fage is my favorite brand), tempeh, tofu, quinoa, almonds, and beans.

CARBOHYDRATES

The carbohydrate is probably the most misunderstood, maligned, and feared macro-nutrient. Thanks to the scores of bogus diet plans and suggestions out there, many people equate eating carbs with getting fat. While eating TOO MANY carbs can make you fat (just as eating too much protein or fat can), carbs are hardly your enemy. They play an essential role in not only muscle growth but in overall body function.

Regardless of what type of carbohydrate you eat—broccoli or apple pie—the body breaks it down into two substances: *glucose* and *glycogen*. Glucose is commonly referred to as "blood sugar," and it's an energy source used by your cells to do the many things they do. Glycogen is a substance stored in the liver and muscles that can be easily converted to glucose for immediate energy. When you lift weights intensely, your muscles burn up their glycogen stores to cope with the overload.

Now, why is broccoli good for you but apple pie isn't? Because your body reacts very differently to broccoli than to apple pie. You've probably heard the terms "simple" and "complex" carbs before and wondered what they meant. You might have also heard of the *glycemic index* and wondered what it was all about.

These things are actually pretty simple. The glycemic index is a numeric system of ranking how quickly carbohydrates are converted into glucose in the body. Carbs are ranked on a scale of 0 to 100 depending on how they affect blood sugar levels once eaten. A GI rating of 55 and under is considered "low GI," 56 to 69 is medium, and 70 and above is high on the index. A "simple" carb is one that converts very quickly (is high on the glycemic index), such as table sugar, honey, and watermelon, while a "complex" carb is one that converts slowly (is low on the glycemic index), such as broccoli, apple, and whole-grain bread.

It's very important to know where the carbs you eat fall on the index, because studies have linked regular consumption of high-GI carbs to increased risk for heart disease, diabetes, and obesity. They do have their uses, though, which we will go over shortly.

FATS

Fats are the densest energy sources available to your body. Each gram of fat contains over twice the calories of a gram of carbohydrate or protein. Healthy fats, such as those found in olive oil, avocados, flax seed oil, many nuts, and other foods are actually an important component to overall health. Fats help your body absorb the other nutrients that you give it, nourish the nervous system, help maintain cell structures, regulate hormone levels, and more.

Saturated fat is a form of fat found mainly in animal products such as meat, dairy products, and egg yolks. Some plant foods, such as coconut oil, palm oil, and palm kernel oil, are also high in saturated fats. While it's commonly believed that eating saturated fat harms your health, recent research has shown this to be untrue[9].

Trans fat is a scientifically modified form of saturated fat that has been engineered to give foods longer shelf lives. Many cheap, packaged foods are full of trans fat (such as run-of-the-mill popcorn, yogurt, and peanut butter), as are many frozen foods (such as frozen pizza, packaged pastries, cakes, etc.). Fried foods are often cooked in trans fat. This type of fat is bad news, and eating too much of it can lead to all kinds of disease and complications. It has no nutritional value for the body and thus should be avoided altogether.

WATER

The human body is about 60% water in adult males and about 70% in adult females. Muscles are about 70% water. That alone tells you how important staying hydrated is to maintaining good health and proper body function. Your body's ability to digest, transport, and absorb nutrients from food is dependent upon proper fluid intake. Water helps prevent injuries in the gym by cushioning joints and other soft-tissue areas. When your body is dehydrated, literally every physiological process is negatively affected.

I really can't stress enough the importance of drinking clean, pure water. It has zero calories, so it will never cause you to gain weight regardless of how much you drink. (You can actually harm your body by drinking too much water, but this would require that you drink several gallons per day.)

The Institute of Medicine reported in 2004 that women should consume about 91 ounces of water—or three-quarters of a gallon—per day, and men should consume about 125 ounces per day (a gallon is 128 ounces).

Now, keep in mind that those numbers include the water found in food. The average person gets about 80% of their water from drinking it and other beverages, and about 20% from the food they eat.

I've been drinking 1-2 gallons of water per day for years now, which is more than the IOM baseline recommendation, but I sweat a fair amount due to exercise and I live in Florida, which surely makes my needs higher. I fill a one-gallon jug at the start of my day and simply make sure that I finish it by dinner time. By the time I go to bed, I'll have drunk a few more glasses.

Make sure the water you drink is filtered, purified water and not tap water. There's a big difference between drinking clean, alkaline water that your body can fully utilize and drinking polluted, acidic junk from the tap or bottle (which is the case with certain brands such as Dasani and Aquafina).

I have a $250 reverse-osmosis filter with a re-mineralization component at home that produces clean, crisp water. A cheaper option is a pitcher with a built-in filter, like those made by Brita and Pur.

VITAMINS AND MINERALS

The importance of vitamins and minerals is unknown to many. Woman will rush to the store to buy the latest super-advanced, "fat-burning" pill that contains a "proprietary blend" of fancy-sounding snake oil compounds, but few of them will pick up a multi-vitamin.

The fact is that your body needs a wide spectrum of vitamins and minerals to carry out the millions of sophisticated functions it performs every day. This is a basic need, like protein, carbohydrates, fats, and water.

Ideally, we'd get all of the vitamins and minerals we need from the food we eat, but this is nearly impossible with the ever-declining quality of American soil and food (even in the world of organic). Thus, we need to supplement our food with vitamin and mineral pills. The easiest way to get all of the essential vitamins and minerals is a good multi-vitamin product.

15

EAT THIS, NOT THAT—
THINNER LEANER STRONGER
VERSION

HAVE YOU SEEN THAT STUPID book, *Eat This, Not That*? Eat a Big Mac that only has 540 calories instead of an Angus Deluxe, which has 750, AND LOSE WEIGHT! Eat a Coldstone Creamery Oreo Crème Ice Cream Sandwich instead of a Sinless Cake 'n Shake Milkshake, and GET SKINNY! Eat your way thin! Lose big without ever stepping foot in the gym!

While that book's meteoric rise to popularity is a sad indictment of people's lack of willpower and ignorance as to how the body actually works, I do have to give the author props for the idea. It was the perfect product for suckers whose idea of losing weight is making their own Banana-Rum Split instead of getting the 1,000 calorie Baskin Robbins version.

Well, I'm going to give you the *Thinner Leaner Stronger* version of *Eat This, Not That*. We're going to look at different types of proteins, carbs, and fats, which you should eat and which you should avoid, and a few more rules of eating that will help you achieve your fitness goals.

TYPES OF PROTEINS

There are two main sources of protein out there: whole food protein and supplement protein.

Whole food protein is, as you guessed, protein that comes from natural food sources, such as beef, chicken, fish, etc. The best forms of whole food protein are chicken, turkey, lean red meat, fish, eggs, and milk. If you're vegetarian, your best options are eggs, low-fat cottage cheese (Organic Valley is my favorite brand), low-fat European style (Greek) yogurt (0% Fage is my favorite), tempeh, tofu, quinoa, almonds, rice, and beans.

While we're on the subject of vegetarianism, some people claim that you must carefully combine your proteins if you're vegetarian or vegan to ensure your body is getting "complete" proteins (all of the amino acids needed to build tissue). This theory and the faulty research it was based on was thoroughly debunked as a myth by the Massachusetts Institute of Technology[10], yet it still hangs around. While it's true that some sources of vegetable protein are lower in certain amino acids than other forms of protein, there is no scientific evidence to prove that they lack them altogether.

Protein supplements are powdered or liquid foods that contain protein from various sources, such as whey (a liquid remaining after milk has been curdled and strained in the process of making cheese), egg, and soy—the three most common sources of supplement protein. There are also great plant-based supplements out there that are a blend of high-quality protein sources such as quinoa, brown rice, peas, hemp, and fruit.

You don't NEED protein supplements to eat well, but it can be impractical for some to try to get all their protein from whole foods. Protein powder is convenient.

Now, there are a few things you should know about eating protein.

First is the subject of how much protein you can absorb in one sitting. Studies relating to this are very contradictory and disputed, mainly because it's a complex subject. Your genetics, metabolism, digestive tract health, lifestyle, and amount of lean mass are all important factors. But in the spirit of keeping things simple, here's what we know: you can eat and properly use a lot of protein in each meal. How much, exactly? Well, your body should have no trouble absorbing upwards of 60 grams in one sitting.

That said, there aren't any benefits of eating this way (I find gorging quite uncomfortable, actually), but it's good to know in case you miss a meal and need to make it up by loading protein into a later meal.

Another thing to know about protein is that different proteins digest at different speeds, and some are better utilized by the body than others. Beef protein, for example, is digested quickly, and 70-80% of what's eaten is utilized by the body (the exact number varies based on what study you read, but they all fall between 70 and 80%). Whey protein is also digested quickly and its "net protein utilization" (the scientific term referring to the body's utilization of the protein) is between 90-95% depending on which study you read. Egg protein digests much slower than whey and beef, and its NPU also falls in the same range as whey.

NPU and digestion speeds are important to know because you want to rely on high-NPU proteins to meet your daily protein requirement, and you want a quick-digesting protein for your post-workout meal, and a slow-digesting protein for your final meal before you go to bed.

I could give you charts and tables of the NPU rates of various proteins, but I'm going to just keep it simple. In order to meet your daily protein requirements, here are your choices:

Whole Food Proteins

Lean meats (beef, pork, chicken, and turkey)

Fish

Eggs

Vegetarian sources noted above

Protein Supplements

Egg

Whey

Casein

High-quality plant-based protein supplements

In case you're wondering why I left soy protein off the list of recommended supplements, it's because of the controversy regarding its effects on our hormones (research has shown that regular consumption of soy can increase estrogen levels[11]). I'm well aware that research has indicated the opposite—that regular soy consumption doesn't have any feminizing effects on men[12]—but I chose to remain on the safe side until further research is done. I also don't like that most soy protein supplements use genetically modified soybeans, but that's a discussion I will go into in a future book.

Now, regarding when to eat slow- or fast-digesting proteins, I recommend eating a fast-digesting protein like whey after working out to quickly spike amino acid levels in your blood and stimulate muscle growth[13.] You should eat a slow-digesting protein like egg or casein thirty minutes before going to bed, as research has shown that this improves muscle recovery[14]. For the rest of your supplement meals, you can do whey or egg. I like to use egg supplements because too much whey tends to bloat me.

TYPES OF CARBOHYDRATES

Your daily carbohydrate intake is vitally important to gain muscle and strength. Carbs fuel your workouts and enable you to properly overload your muscles, and they play a crucial role in pre- and post-workout meals.

That being said, the majority of carbs eaten by most people are not only unhealthy because of genetically modified ingredients and heavy processing, but are also pretty high on the GI, which makes them even worse for the body.

Below is a list of common snack foods with corresponding average GI scores. The GI scores vary a bit from brand to brand, but not by much.

(The following information is sourced from the University of Sydney, the University of Harvard, and Livestrong.com.)

FOOD	GI
White bread bagel	72
Corn chips	63
Pretzels	83
Breakfast cereal like Cornflakes, Special K, Raisin Bran, etc.	72-84
Candy bar	62-78
Wheat or corn cracker	67-87
Rye cracker	64
Rice cake	78
Popcorn	72
White rice	64
Pizza	80
Whole wheat bread	71
White bread	70
Baguette	95
English muffin (white bread)	77
Baked potato	85
Instant oatmeal	83
Coca Cola	63

If you're a little dismayed to find many of your favorite snacks on that list, I understand. Unfortunately, these foods simply can't be eaten often if you want to have high, stable energy levels, and if you want to have a lean, vital body.

Regardless of how many carbs you need to eat per day (based on what you're trying to accomplish with your body), there's a simple rule to follow regarding high-, medium- and low-glycemic carbs.

Eat carbs in the medium-high range of the glycemic index (70-90 is a good rule of thumb) about thirty minutes before you train and within thirty minutes of finishing your workout. (We will work out the exact amounts for you soon.)

The reason you want some carbs before training is that you need the energy for your training. The reason you want them after is that your muscles are starved for glycogen, and by replacing it quickly, you actually help your body maintain an anabolic state and not lose muscle tissue.

My favorite pre- and post-workout carbs are bananas and rice milk, but other good choices are unprocessed foods on the high-GI list above, such as baked potato, white rice, instant oatmeal, and fruits that are above 60 on the glycemic index, such as cantaloupe, pineapple, watermelon, dates, apricots, and figs. Some people recommend eating foods high in table sugar (sucrose) after working out because it's high on the GI, but I stay away from processed sugar as much as possible.

All other carbs you eat should be in the middle or low end of the glycemic index (60 and below is a good rule of thumb). It's really that simple. If you follow this rule, you'll avoid so many problems that others suffer from due to energy highs and lows, and eventually even disease, that come with regularly eating high-GI carbs.

Below are some examples of tasty, healthy carbs that you can include in your diet:

FOOD	GI
Multi-grain bread	43
Multi-grain muffin	45
Whole grain sourdough bread	48
Basmati rice	43
Brown rice	55
Apple	38
Yam	37
Black beans	30

Peanuts	14
Almonds	10
Strawberries	40
Blackberries	32
Oatmeal	58
Orange	42

Forget stuff like sugar, white bread, processed, low-quality whole wheat bread, junk cereals, muffins, white pasta, crackers, waffles, and corn flakes. I wouldn't even recommend eating these types of processed foods as pre- or post-workout carbs because they're just not good for your body.

Even certain fruits, such as watermelon and dates, are bad everyday snack foods because of where they fall on the glycemic index. If you're unsure about a carb you like, look it up to see where it falls on the glycemic index. If it's above 60, just leave it out of your meals that aren't immediately before or after working out.

TYPES OF FATS

Getting enough healthy fats every day is pretty simple. The rule works like this:

- Keep your intake of saturated fats relatively low (below 10% of your total calories). Saturated fat is found in foods like meat, dairy, eggs, coconut oil, bacon fat, and lard. If a fat is solid at room temperature, it's a saturated fat.

- Completely avoid trans fats, which are the worst type of dietary fat. Trans fats are found in processed foods, such as cookies, cakes, fries, and donuts. Any food that contains "hydrogenated oil" or "partially hydrogenated oil" likely contains trans fats, so just don't eat it. (Sure, having a cheat here and there that contains trans fats won't harm anything, but you definitely don't want to eat them regularly.)

- Get much of your fats from unsaturated sources, such as olive oil, nuts, peanut oil, avocados, flax seed oil, safflower oil, sesame oil, or cottonseed oil. If a fat is liquid at room temperature, it's an unsaturated fat.

SODIUM

The average American's diet is so over-saturated with sodium it makes my head spin.

The Institute of Medicine recommends 1,500 milligrams of sodium per day as the adequate intake level for most adults, and an upper limit of 2,300 mg per day. Most people eat a lot more than this, however. According to the CDC, the average American aged 2 and up eats 3,436 milligrams of sodium per day.

Over-consumption of sodium is surprisingly easy. A teaspoon of table salt contains a whopping 2,300 mg of sodium. Yup, you read that right—one teaspoon of table salt per day is the recommended upper limit of sodium intake (and that's why I use potassium chloride—a salt substitute—instead of table salt).

I recommend looking over your sodium intake and bringing it down to the IOM's adequate intake level, as chronic high sodium intake is not only bad for how you look, but can lead to high blood pressure and even heart disease.

It's also worth noting that ensuring your body gets enough potassium is important, as it helps balance fluids in the cells (sodium sucks water in, potassium pumps it out). According to the Institute of Medicine, we should be consuming sodium and potassium at about a 1:2 ratio, with 4,700 mg per day as the adequate intake of potassium for adults.

There are many natural sources of potassium, such as all meats and fish; vegetables like broccoli, peas, tomatoes, sweet potatoes, and beans; dairy products; and nuts. You can also buy potas¬sium tablets that you can supplement with, if necessary.

THE BOTTOM LINE

You may find this chapter a bit hard to swallow (no pun intended). Some people have a really hard time giving up their unhealthy eating habits (sugar and junk food can be pretty addictive). That being said, consider the following benefits of following the advice in this chapter:

1. If this is a completely new way of eating for you, I *guarantee* you'll feel better than you have in a *long* time. You won't have energy highs and lows. You won't feel lethargic. You won't have that mental fogginess that comes with being stuffed full of unhealthy food every day.

2. You will appreciate "bad" food so much more when you only have it once or twice per week. You'd be surprised how much better a

dessert tastes when you haven't had one in a week. (You may also be surprised that junk food that you loved in the past no longer tastes good.)

3. You will actually come to enjoy healthy foods. I *promise*. Even if they don't taste good to you at first, just groove in the routine, and soon you'll crave brown rice and fruit instead of doughnuts and bread. Your body will adapt.

Don't discount the importance of what I covered in this chapter. The types of proteins, carbs, and fats that you eat will not only determine your gains but will also dictate how you look. Eat poorly, and you'll look bloated and puffy. Eat well, and you'll look lean and hard. It's really that simple.

16

HOW TO PLAN YOUR MEALS TO MAXIMIZE YOUR GAINS

MANY PEOPLE'S MEAL PLANS ARE engineered for getting fat. They skip breakfast, eat a junk food lunch, come home famished, have a big dinner with some dessert, and then munch on chips or popcorn while watching TV at night. This is exactly how you ruin your metabolism and pack on layers of ugly fat.

In this chapter, I want to discuss the basics of how to structure your meals each day.

MACRO-NUTRIENT PLANNING

PROTEIN

Ensuring you get enough protein every day is vital to building muscle and staying lean. While the science of how often you should eat protein is a bit hazy, we know that you don't have to eat protein on a rigid schedule (every so many hours). What matters most is that you get enough by the end of each day.

That said, I like to eat protein every 3-5 hours simply because it's filling. I do 4-6 servings of protein per day, which allows me to keep the meals smaller (which again is more enjoyable, I think).

CARBOHYDRATES

Much of your daily carbohydrates will come before and after training, when your body needs them most.

I'd also like to address the subject of eating carbs within several hours of going to bed. This advice has been kicking around the health and fitness world for quite some time, but usually with the wrong explanation.

There's no scientific evidence that eating carbs at night or before bed will lead to gaining fat, but it may *hinder* fat loss. How?

The insulin created by the body to process and absorb carbs eaten stops the use of fat as an energy source. Your body naturally burns the most fat while sleeping, and so going to sleep with elevated insulin levels can theoretically interfere with fat loss.

Related to this is the fact that studies have indicated that the production and processing of insulin interferes with the production and processing of growth hormone[15, 16], which has powerful fat-burning properties. Your body naturally produces much of its growth hormone while sleeping, so again, if your insulin levels are elevated when you go to sleep, your growth hormone production may suffer, which in turn would rob you of its fat-burning benefits.

Research in this area is currently lacking, but when I'm cutting, I don't see any need to eat a lot of carbs before bed, so I restrict my intake after dinner. I want my insulin to be as close to baseline as possible when I go to sleep.

FATS

You can spread your fats throughout the day. I like to start my day with 1-2 tablespoons of Udo's oil (a great 3-6-9 blend), but you don't have to buy this if you don't want to. You can simply stick to the sources of healthy fat given earlier.

THE PRE-WORKOUT MEAL: 30 – 20 – 20

About 30 minutes before training, you want to eat about 20 grams of high-GI carbs and about 20 grams of fast-digesting protein (such as whey).

The carbs will not only give you energy to fuel your workout, they will trigger the release of insulin, which counteracts the effects of cortisol and, according to a study done at the University of Oklahoma, increases blood flow to the muscles and protein synthesis[17].

The protein will get amino acids into your bloodstream, immediately available for repair as you start to break down the muscle fibers by lifting weights.

THE POST-WORKOUT MEAL

Many people are surprised to learn how important eating a post-workout meal is.

Research has shown shown that eating carbs and protein after weight training leads to greater massmuscle growth, and improved exercise performance in subsequent workouts[18].

When you finish training, your body will absorb glucose, glycogen, and amino acids at a higher rate than normal. If you fail to eat during this "window," you waste an opportunity to speed up your progress toward your goals.

Therefore, it's important to eat within an hour or so of finishing your weight training, and to eat a substantial amount of carbs, and a moderate amount of protein. For most women, this is about 50 grams of medium-to-high-GI carbs, and 20-30 grams of protein. (Don't worry—we will work out your exact numbers soon.)

It's also worth noting that the above recommendations are for after your weight training, not cardio. You don't have to load carbs after cardio, because it doesn't deplete glycogen stores like weightlifting does. The exception is if you're engaging in long (1+ hour), intense cardio, involving plenty of sprinting or other anaerobic activity. That said, I like to have some protein before cardio to minimize muscle breakdown.

PRE-SLEEP MEAL

A slow-digesting protein should be the last meal of the night, and should be consumed immediately before going to bed. Research has shown that this keeps amino acids elevated while you sleep, which can then be used to continue to repair your muscles while you sleep[19]. This speeds your muscle recovery.

I like egg protein powder or 0% fat Greek yogurt or low-fat cottage cheese for my pre-sleep protein, but casein is another common choice.

IT'S TIME TO CHEAT!

Many people struggling with diets talk about "cheat days." The idea is that if you're good during the week, you can go buck wild on the weekends and somehow not gain fat. Well, unless you have a very fast metabolism, that's not how it works. If you follow a strict diet and exercise, you can expect to lose 1-2 pounds per week. If you get too crazy, you can gain it right back over a weekend.

There are much smarter ways to go about cheating.

The first important point is to think in cheat *meals*, not *days*. No sensible diet should include entire days of overeating, but a single bout of overeating per week is actually advisable when you're dieting to lose weight.

Why?

Well, there's the psychological boost, which keeps you happy and motivated, which ultimately makes sticking to your diet easier[20].

But there's also a physiological boost.

Studies on overfeeding (the scientific term for binging on food) show that doing so can boost your metabolic rate by anywhere from 3–10%[21]. While this sounds good, it actually doesn't mean much when you consider that you would need to eat anywhere from a few hundred to a few thousand *extra* calories in a day to achieve this effect, thus negating the calorie-related benefits.

More important, however, are the effects cheating has on the hormone *leptin*, which regulates hunger, your metabolic rate, appetite, motivation, and libido, as well as serving other functions in your body.

When you're in a caloric deficit and lose body fat, your leptin levels drop[22]. This, in turn, causes your metabolic rate to slow down, your appetite to increase, your motivation to wane, and your mood to sour.

When you boost your leptin levels, this can have positive effects on fat oxidation, thyroid activity, mood, and even testosterone levels. What you really want from a cheat meal is a leptin boost.

Eating carbohydrates is the most effective way[23]. Second to that is eating protein (high-protein meals also raise your metabolic rate[24]). Dietary fats aren't very effective at increasing leptin levels, and alcohol actually inhibits it[25].

How many cheat meals you should eat per week depends on what you're trying to accomplish.

When you're bulking, two or three cheat meals per week is totally fine.

When you're cutting, you can have one cheat meal per week, and I recommend that you make it a "re-feed meal," which I'll explain in full in the next chapter.

EATING ON YOUR OFF DAYS

Don't worry about lowering your calories for your off days (days that you don't train on). While it might seem to make sense as you're burning less calories on those days, practically speaking, it won't make a difference if you reduce them or not.

The only change I make on off days is I don't eat my high-carb post-workout meal, which is my breakfast as I train early in the morning. Instead, I usually have the same amount of calories and carbs with a hot cereal like oatmeal and a protein such as eggs, a protein shake, fat-free yogurt, and so forth.

THE BOTTOM LINE

Building a great body requires great eating habits, and you now know what that means: eating enough calories, protein, carbohydrates, and fats on the right eating schedule and drinking enough water, ensuring that your body has everything it needs to adapt to the intense training that you subject it to.

17

YOUR *THINNER LEANER STRONGER* DIET PLAN

IN ORDER TO DIET PROPERLY, you need to know how to determine how many calories to eat each day and how many of those calories should be from proteins, carbs, and fats.

Well, that's what we're going to cover in this chapter: how to calculate your exact diet requirements for losing weight and "maintaining," which is eating so you can slowly build muscle without gaining any fat.

There are many formulas and methods out there for calculating caloric and macro targets. Some are based on the idea that you should eat based on your target weight, not where you currently are. While I've found these methods workable, they require that you know your body fat percentage, which can be a bit of problem. Hand-held electrical devices that claim to measure body fat percentage can be horribly inaccurate, as can scales that "measure" body fat levels. Taking measurements and entering them into an online body fat percentage calculator of some kind will give wildly inaccurate results in almost all cases.

Thus, the method for calculating your diet that I'm going to share is based on your current body weight and goal (lose weight, or slowly build muscle while gaining little-to-no fat). It's very simple and workable.

In case you're interested in knowing your body fat percentage, most experts agree that hydrostatic testing, DEXA x-ray, and BodPod testing are the most accurate methods of determining body fat percentage. The downside, however, is inconvenience and cost.

Therefore, I recommend that you get a good fat caliper. When you learn how to test properly with this simple device, you will get very accurate measurements. I recommend a good, cheap caliper in the bonus report at the end of this book and on my website, www.muscleforlife.com, along with other equipment such as supplements, gloves, shoes, and more.

DIETING FOR MAXIMUM FAT LOSS

Losing fat simply requires that you reduce your daily caloric intake, and as you'll see, most of the calories you cut from your diet come from reducing your carbs.

Losing weight requires more precision than maintaining as you're looking to keep your calories at a very specific level that will allow you to steadily lose fat with minimal strength and muscle loss. If you eat a bit too much every day, you'll hinder your fat loss, and if you eat a bit too little, you'll risk losing muscle.

In case you've never done it before, I want to warn you that the first week or two of dieting to lose weight is a bit rough. You're going to be hungry, and you're going to crave carbs. It's just the way it is. Stay strong, however, and you'll find it much easier from week two on. By week four or five, you won't even mind it anymore.

CALCULATING YOUR WEIGHT LOSS DIET

You will first calculate a starting point for your diet and then adjust as needed. You've nailed it when you lose 1-2 pounds per week with little or no strength loss. If you're losing a lot of strength, you're also losing muscle (which means your calories are too low).

Here's how to calculate your starting point:

- Eat 1.2 grams of protein per pound of body weight per day

- Eat 1 gram of carbs per pound of body weight per day

- Eat .2 grams of healthy fat per pound of body weight per day (1 gram per 5 pounds of body weight per day)

That's where you start. For a 140 lb woman, it would look like this:

- 168 grams of protein per day

- 140 grams of carbs per day

- 28 grams of fat per day

This would be about 1,484 calories per day, which is a good starting point for a 140 lb woman.

If you're obese (over 25% body for men and 30% for women), your formula is slightly different:

- .8 grams of protein per pound of body weight

- .7 grams of carbs per pound of body weight

- .3 grams of fat per pound of body weight

For a 175 lb woman, it would look like this (note that I'm rounding these numbers down):

- 140 grams of protein per day

- 120 grams of carbs per day

- 50 grams of fat per day

This comes to about 1,500 calories per day, and is a perfect place for a 175 lb woman to start losing weight.

Now, eating this much protein feels unusual at first for most women, but eating a lot of protein is actually vital to both building and retaining muscle, and losing weight. Studies, such as the University of Illinois study published in 2005 have shown that, when combined with exercise, high-protein diets help women retain muscle mass, and even, strangely enough, lose more weight in their midsection.

If you find it very hard to keep your fats this low, you can tweak the diet by reducing your carbs by 50 grams each day and increasing your fats by about 20 grams.

THE DANGER OF HIDDEN CALORIES

A huge, killer diet trap that many people fall into is they eat a lot of "hidden calories" throughout the day and then wonder why they aren't losing weight. Hidden calories are those that you don't realize are there, such as the following:

- The two tablespoons of olive oil used to cook your chicken breast (240 calories)

- The two tablespoons of mayonnaise in your homemade chicken salad (200 calories)

- The three cubes of feta cheese on your salad (140 calories)

- The three tablespoons of cream in your coffee (80 calories)

- The two pats of butter with your toast (70 calories)

Hidden calories are the number one reason why people don't get results from properly calculated and planned diets. They just eat more than they're supposed to, usually by eating out at restaurants, ordering what they think are low-calorie menu items.

When you're dieting to lose weight, you'll be running on a 500-600 calorie deficit every day, so as you can see, there's little margin for error.

If you eat 400 hidden calories and thus only really have a 100-200 calorie deficit at the end of the day, you won't lose much weight. It's that simple. It might seem paranoid to be careful about how many tablespoons of ketchup you eat in a day, but if you watch your calories that closely when dieting to lose weight, you are *guaranteed* to get results. Your body WILL get lean.

The best way to avoid hidden calories is to prepare your food yourself, so you know exactly what went into it (for most this just means preparing a lunch to bring to the office, as breakfast and dinner are usually eaten at home).

SIGNS THAT YOU HAVE YOUR DIET RIGHT OR WRONG

After 2-3 weeks of sticking to your diet, you should assess how it's going. Weight loss isn't the only criterion to consider when deciding if your diet is right or wrong, however.

You should judge your progress based on the following criteria:

Your weight (did it go down, up, or stay the same?)

Your clothes (do they feel looser, tighter, or the same?)

The mirror (do you look thinner, fatter, or the same?)

Your energy levels (do you feel energized, tired, or somewhere in between?)

Your strength (is it going up, down, or staying about the same?)

Your sleep (are you exhausted by the end of the night, do you have trouble winding down, or has nothing changed?)

Let's talk about each point briefly.

WEIGHT

If your weight is going up, you're eating too much. Even if you're new to weight lifting and thus will be building muscle, it won't be more than the 1-2 pounds of fat per week that you should be losing.

If your weight is the same after several weeks of dieting, you may be eating too much, but you may just be building muscle to replace the weight of the fat lost (and you'll know it by your clothing and mirror, which we're going to talk about).

If your weight is going down, then that's a good sign, although there are other factors to consider to ensure you're not eating too little, which brings other problems (you'll see in a minute).

YOUR CLOTHES

If your jeans feel a bit looser and your tops a bit looser in the shoulders, that's a good sign. If your weight also hasn't changed, then you should count yourself lucky—you've built muscle and lost fat!

YOUR MIRROR

Although it can be tough to see changes in our bodies due to seeing them every day, you should definitely notice a difference after several weeks of dieting to lose weight. You should look less puffy and visibly leaner.

If you don't, chances are your weight hasn't changed either, or has gone up, and your jeans aren't feeling looser. This is a clear sign that you're still eating too much.

If you look thinner in the mirror and your jeans are looser, yet your weight hasn't changed, then chances are you've built muscle to replace the weight of the fat you lost, or your muscles are holding additional water, or it's a bit of both. Either way, so long as you're getting leaner, carry on.

YOUR ENERGY LEVELS

You should never feel starved and running on empty when dieting to lose weight. Depending on how you ate before starting the weight loss process, you may feel a little hungry for the first week or two, but after that, you should feel comfortable throughout the day.

In terms of energy, we all have high- and low-energy days, but if you're having more lows than usual, then chances are you're not eating enough.

YOUR STRENGTH

If you're new to weight training and start with dieting to lose weight, your strength should go up week after week. If it isn't, this can be caused by under-eating, by not training properly, or by not resting properly.

If you're an experienced weightlifter, it's not uncommon to see a minor loss in strength due to cutting carbs, but it shouldn't be more than 5% or so. If your strength drops by 10% or more, chances are you're under-eating.

SLEEP

If you're dead tired by bed time, that's not necessarily a bad sign. This is common when people start training correctly.

What's important, however, is that you sleep long and deeply. If your heart is beating quickly at night and you're anxious, tossing and turning in bed, and if you wake up more often at night, you might be overtraining, or under-eating.

MENSTRUAL CYCLE

Although you can't tell this within only three weeks of starting your weight loss diet, you should know that if your cycles become longer or unpredictable, you might be under-eating, which can mess with your hormones.

On the other hand, if your cycles are normally unpredictable and they become regular, this is probably a good sign that you're eating well.

SUMMARY

If, based on the above criteria, you suspect you're eating too much, all you need to do is cut your calories by 200 per day and see if that fixes it within the next two weeks. To cut these calories, simply cut your carbs by 50 grams per day. Don't eat less protein or fats.

If you suspect you're eating too little, add 200 calories in carbs per day and see if this stabilizes your strength (it should).

As a note, you should adjust your calories down by about 200 for every 15 pounds that you lose. You should subtract these calories by reducing carbs (reduce by 50 grams per day).

GENERAL RULES FOR DIETING TO LOSE WEIGHT

Weight loss requires that you be very precise with how much you eat. You want to walk a fine line of running at enough of a calorie deficit to lose fat but not dropping too low, which would cause muscle and strength loss.

When I'm dieting to lose weight, I try to be within 50-100 calories of my daily target. If I'm a little higher, so be it. If I'm a little lower, that's okay too. It really just depends on what types of foods I feel like eating. Then I see how my body responds and adjust as needed.

Eat 30-40% of your daily carbs in your post-workout meal. Make sure to have the rest eaten by the end of dinner. If you train at night, what I've found workable is cutting my normal post-workout carbs in half, and spreading the remaining half throughout the day.

For instance, if my post-workout meal was supposed to include 80 grams of carbs, I'd do 40 grams after training, and eat the remaining 40 grams earlier in the day. You should have no trouble losing weight as long as you get everything else right.

Stick to lean white-meat proteins such as chicken, fish, turkey, and eggs. When I'm dieting to lose weight, I do 1-2 servings of red meat per week. If you're a vegetarian, you'll just have to watch your fat intake.

CHEATING WHEN DIETING TO LOSE WEIGHT

There's a great method of cheating when dieting to lose weight that not only satisfies your cravings, but actually helps preserve your muscle and maintain your strength. It's known as "re-feeding."

The theory is simple: When you start running your body on a caloric deficit, evolution has programmed it to adjust in several ways to ensure it won't die of starvation (an overreaction of course, but old habits die hard).

Metabolism slows down, hunger increases, and the sacrifice of muscle for energy begins. Production of the thyroid hormone T3, which works together with T4 to regulate metabolism, drops, and cortisol stays in your system longer (interfering with muscle synthesis). Testosterone production also drops.

On top of all of that, intense weightlifting five days per week thoroughly depletes glycogen levels in the muscles, and low glycogen levels means less strength and muscle growth.

This is basically a nightmare scenario for anyone who is trying to get lean and keep their muscle. So, what can you do about it?

Plan one day per week where you eat double your normal amount of carbs. This will replenish glycogen stores in the muscles and kick the thyroid into gear. It will also spike leptin levels, the benefits of which you learned earlier in the book. I recommend you plan it on a day which is followed by a training day. Many people plan it for the day before they train their lagging muscle group(s) because the boost in carbs results in higher energy in the gym.

You can pack the extra carbs into one carb-laden meal if you want—one where you eat 0.5 to 1 gram of carbs per pound of body weight—or you can spread it out over two or three meals during the day.

I like to eat about 100 grams of carbs for breakfast (pancakes!), and another 100 or so at lunch (usually whole-wheat pasta), and then add one extra piece of fruit in my afternoon snack. That, combined with my normal carbs for the day, bumps me up to about 400 grams for the day, which is a perfect re-feed.

Now, your numbers will be less, of course, but the idea is simple. Just double your carbs one day per week.

A proper re-feed not only won't cause any fat storage, but will also prevent your body from getting sucked into the dwindling spiral I explained earlier.

If you'd rather not re-feed, that's okay too. You can simply do one cheat meal per week when dieting to lose weight. A cheat meal is one where you eat more than you normally would. I don't recommend gorging, but don't be afraid to enjoy it, either. Go out with friends, eat some pasta, have some dessert, and don't feel guilty. You've earned it.

FIGURING OUT WHAT TO ACTUALLY EAT AND WHEN

Many people struggling with losing weight feel like they're not eating a lot, but when they track their meals and actually look at the calories, it's always too much. This is easily remedied by planning out meals ahead of time so you know that you're eating the right amount.

So, how do you translate numeric requirements of calories, protein, carbs, and fat into actual meals? Simple! You create meals using a food nutrition database, like CalorieKing.com or caloriecount.about.com (my two favorites).

It's very important that you work out exact meals and stick to them because, as you know, all it takes to kill your fat loss is a few hundred hidden calories per day.

I recommend using a spreadsheet to work this out, and the simplest way to do it is to list out, meal by meal, a full day's worth of food that you can easily prepare and stick to. List out the calories, protein, carbs, and fat of each food for each meal, totaling the numbers as you go. Tweak things as needed until you have one day's worth of food that meets your caloric and macro-nutritional needs.

Then, create substitute meals that you can choose when you want something different for breakfast, lunch, dinner, or other meals. I like to have a few options for breakfast, lunch, and dinner and find that as long as I rotate them every few days, I never get sick of any of them.

Let's work out a daily meal plan for a 150 lb woman who wants to lose a bit of weight. For the purpose of this meal plan, let's say she lifts weights at night. I'm going to include a few meals from my cookbook, *The Shredded Chef*. If you want to check out the recipes, snag the free bonus report offered at the end of the book (or the cookbook).

Target Daily Protein: 180 grams

Target Daily Carbs: 150 grams

Target Daily Fats: 30 grams

Target Daily Calories: 1590

Meal #1 (8:15 am)

1 serving of Veggie Egg & Cheese Scramble

273 calories

32 grams of protein

8 grams of carbs

9 grams of fat

Meal #2 (10:30 am)

1 cup of low-fat cottage cheese

1 medium orange

265 calories

30 grams of protein

16 grams of carbs

4 grams of fat

Meal #3 (12:30 pm)

1 serving of Quick & Easy Protein Salad

272 calories

24 grams of protein

31 grams of carbs

5 grams of fat

Meal #4 (3:30 pm)

1 Strawberry Banana Protein Bar

199 calories

22 grams of protein

16 grams of carbs

5 grams of fat

Meal #5 (pre-workout 5:30 pm)

1 scoop of protein powder in water

1 medium orange

190 calories

30 grams of protein

16 grams of carbs

0 grams of fat

Meal #6 (post-workout 7:00 pm)

1 serving of Graham-Coated Tilapia

1 apple

320 calories

25 grams of protein

35 grams of carbs

10 grams of fat

Meal #7 (10:30 pm)

20 grams of casein or egg protein

80 calories

20 grams of protein

0 grams of carbs

1 gram of fat

SUMMARY

This meal plan provides 1,599 calories, 183 grams of protein, 122 grams of carbs, and 34 grams of fat. which is a great place for our 150 lb friend to start losing weight.

Remember that the numbers you calculate are *targets*—you don't have to wrack your brains trying to juggle foods or ingredients so you meet them exactly or within a tiny margin.

DIETING TO MAINTAIN

You diet to maintain once you're happy with your leanness and want to slowly build and strengthen your muscles without adding any fat.

Now, don't think of "maintaining" as "staying the same." I think you should always have the goal of getting at least a little stronger every month, and most women always want to improve the shape or look of certain areas of their bodies. Always set goals and be looking to improve. Don't just try to stay the same because things tend to either get better or get worse.

CALCULATING YOUR MAINTENANCE DIET

Here's how you determine your starting point:

- Eat 1 gram of protein per pound of body weight per day

- Eat 1.5 grams of carbs per pound of body weight per day

- Eat 1 gram of healthy fats per 4 pounds of body weight per day

That's where you start. For a 130 lb woman, it would look like this:

- 130 grams of protein per day

- 195 grams of carbs per day

- 32 grams of fat per day

That's about 1,600 calories per day, which should work for making slow, steady muscle and strength gains without any fat added along the way.

GENERAL RULES FOR MAINTAINING

You should create a daily meal plan and stick to it each day. If you're 50-100 calories over your target, don't sweat it.

You can plan a variety, of course, but make sure that you know exactly what's going into your body each day.

You can still cheat once or twice per week, and you don't have to worry about re-feeding as your carbs are high enough.

Eat at least 30% of your daily carbs in your post-workout meal, but feel free to go higher if you'd like. Remember that the post-workout feeding "window" is a great time to load in the carbs.

SIGNS THAT YOU HAVE YOUR DIET RIGHT OR WRONG

You should evaluate your progress by the same criteria given for judging your weight loss diet.

When maintaining, your weight is less of an indicator of progress than when dieting to lose weight. You can lose a little fat and build a little muscle each week, and your weight can stay more or less the same. Your weight can go up if you build a little muscle but don't lose any fat, and it can go down if you lose a little fat or muscle due to not eating enough.

You should be getting a little stronger each week, and you should notice little positive changes in the mirror and in how your clothes fit. If, after several weeks of following your maintenance diet, your jeans are getting tighter and you look flabbier, then you're eating too much.

You should have good energy levels and should be sleeping well. If your energy levels are low and you're not sleeping well, you might be eating too little, or you might be eating too much of the wrong types of food (too many high-GI carbs or too much trans fats, for instance).

If you suspect you're eating too much, cut 200 calories from your daily target by reducing your carbs by 50 grams per day, and see if that fixes it after a couple of weeks of assessment. If it doesn't, cut further.

If you suspect you're not eating enough, add 200 calories per day by bumping your carbs or fats up (remember, carbs have 4 calories per gram, and fats have 9).

BODY COMPOSITION IS MORE IMPORTANT THAN BODY WEIGHT

Women are so indoctrinated into caring about their weight over everything else that they can be a bit confused by their progress on the *Thinner Leaner Stronger* program.

Unless they're starting out very lean (15% body fat or under), it's very common for women to start on this program and actually build muscle while losing fat. On the scale, this can look like little progress is being made, but when they look at what's happening in the gym and in the mirror, they're clearly progressing.

A great example of this is a friend of mine who has been training with me for about ten months now. When he started, he was just over 220 lbs and about 23% body fat. Within the first three months of training, his strength had nearly doubled across the board, and he had muscle to show for the first time in his life...but he was *twenty* pounds lighter than when he started (which can be quite disconcerting for us guys, as we want to get bigger and stronger, and we equate that with weighing more). This was all fat loss, of course—his body fat tested at around 14%.

Now, seven months later, he has gained over twenty pounds of muscle, putting him back at the same weight as when he started, but his body composition is completely different, and people can't believe the transformation.

So if you're not already lean and fit, don't fret if your weight isn't changing but your strength is going up, your muscles are visually getting tighter, and you're losing fat. Listen to the scale, but let your mirror and weights have the final say.

THE BOTTOM LINE

I know it's a lot to take in all at once, but I have good news. You've just learned everything you'll ever need to know about dieting. You'll never struggle with building muscle or losing fat again if you just follow what you've read in the last few chapters. Feel free to re-read this section of the book a couple of times to let everything really sink in.

Let's now tackle training and look at how to get the most out of our time in the gym each day.

18

THE *THINNER LEANER STRONGER* TRAINING FORMULA

MANY TRAINING PROGRAMS TOUTED in the magazines and infomercials are the same. They want you to use a bunch of machines and maybe some light free weights, and do a bunch of reps. The free weight exercises usually rely on dumbbells, and usually isolate muscles like the biceps, triceps, and shoulders.

While this type of training is better than nothing, there are much better ways to spend your time and energy.

Ironically, machines became a staple of gyms not because they're particularly effective, but they're inviting. They don't look nearly as intimidating as hunks and bars of iron. They're easier to manipulate and, in some cases, you have a reduced risk of injury.

While some machines are useful, such as the cable setup, the majority are inferior to dumbbell and barbell exercises in terms of producing stronger, better developed muscles. Therefore, the *Thinner Leaner Stronger* program will focus on free weights, and not on machines.

When women do use free weights, they usually do isolation exercises. This type of workout comes from the world of men's bodybuilding, in which guys spend hours in the gym each day sculpting each muscle fiber in their bodies for competitive shows. As you can imagine, workouts derived from this style of training are hardly optimal for women that want to look lean and athletic.

The *Thinner Leaner Stronger* program is built around compound exercises—exercises like the Squat, Deadlift, Military Press, Bench Press, and many others. These are the exercises that give you the most bang for your buck—the most total-body strengthening and conditioning for the time and effort.

The *Thinner Leaner Stronger* weight training method follows a formula that looks like this:

$$1 - 2 \mid 8 - 10 \mid 12 \mid 1 - 2 \mid 45 - 60 \mid 5 - 7 \mid 8 - 10$$

No, that isn't a secret code that you have to break. Let's go through this formula one piece at a time.

1-2
TRAIN 1-2 MUSCLE GROUPS PER DAY

You will be training one or two major muscle groups per workout (per day). Your workouts will be one of three types: a workout that trains only one major muscle group (such as chest or legs), a workout that trains one major group and one minor group (such as back and abs), or a workout that trains two minor groups (such as biceps and triceps).

Thinner Leaner Stronger is laid out like this for a couple of reasons. First, it's simply not possible to fully train two major muscle groups in one workout that is under an hour (and you're about to learn why you want your training sessions to be 45-60 minutes long). The second reason is a psychological one. By training only one major muscle group per day, you will be able to give it 100% focus and intensity and train it hard.

8-10
DO SETS OF 8-10 REPS FOR NEARLY ALL EXERCISES

You will be doing 8-10 repetitions per set on virtually *all exercises* (the only exception to this is when training abs, for which I recommend using weight that allows you to do 15-20 reps).

What is meant by doing 8-10 reps? It means that you should use weights that are light enough to allow you to get at least 8 reps, but also heavy enough to prevent you from doing more than 10 reps. If you find you can't do at least 8 reps on an exercise, the weight is too heavy; conversely, if you find you can do more than 10 reps, the weight is too light.

When you can do a set of 10 reps with perfect form, you should add weight to your next set—5 pounds for dumbbell exercises, and 10 pounds for barbell exercises. This should allow you to do 8 reps on your next set, and you build your strength from there over the next few weeks. If adding 10 pounds is too much (if you can't get at least 8 reps on your next set), drop it to a 5-pound increase.

This style of training will probably be new to you, as many weightlifting programs for women call for using extremely light weight. As you now know, however, that this style of training does very little to improve your strength and muscle size and definition. By training with weights heavy enough to limit you to 8-10 reps, however, and by progressively increasing your weights over time, you'll be able to dramatically improve both your strength and muscle shape and tone.

So be ready for a challenge. Be ready to push yourself. Your workouts should feel like work. You don't have to go to absolute failure every set (the point where you simply can't do another rep no matter how hard you try), but your final rep should be a *struggle* without having to sacrifice form.

12

DO 12 WORKING SETS PER MUSCLE GROUP

Your workouts will consist of 12 "working" sets per muscle group trained. A working set is your challenging, 8-10 rep, muscle-building set, as opposed to a warm-up set, which we'll soon go over.

Regardless of which exercises you do, you'll never do more than 12 sets for any individual muscle group.

This might be a shock to some. All too often I see people pounding away on a muscle group, doing 20, 25, or even 30 sets of lifting. This is overtraining, and it's not only a huge waste of time but a huge waste of *muscle*—both potential and existing. The body can't effectively repair that much damage to the muscle fibers, and the result can actually be *shrinkage*.

12 working sets is the sweet spot for total training volume for each muscle group given the weights you'll be handling. By doing 12 working sets per muscle group, you not only fully and deeply stimulate the muscles you're training, but you can keep your workouts in the ideal time frame of 45-60 minutes.

1-2

REST 1-2 MINUTES IN BETWEEN SETS

When you lift weights, many physiological activities take place to enable you to perform the exercise. For a muscle to contract, it requires cellular energy, oxygen, certain chemical reactions, and many other molecular processes. As you perform each rep, you deplete your muscles' capacity to contract forcefully.

Sufficient recovery time in between sets is what allows you to repeat this process enough to achieve the optimum amount of muscle overload to stimulate and force new growth. Basically, the whole point of resting between sets is to prepare your muscles to lift maximum weight in the next set.

The in-between-set recovery period should last about 1-2 minutes. This amount of time allows your muscles to restore their maximum lifting potentials by replenishing energy stores and flushing out unwanted chemical byproducts of the previous set.

Some days you'll feel energized and quicker on recovery, and other days you'll feel a bit slower. The important point is that you give yourself enough time in between sets to be able to lift the maximum amount of weight in each set. If one minute is all you need, great; if you need the full two minutes, that's okay too.

Don't, however, drag out rest times to 5 or 6 minutes or beyond. This drags out the whole workout and kills intensity. The test isn't whether you WANT to do the next set or not; it's whether your body's heart rate has come down since the last set and you feel like you have the energy to do another set.

45-60

TRAIN FOR 45-60 MINUTES

If your workouts are going longer than an hour, something is wrong. You should be able to finish every *Thinner Leaner Stronger* workout in about 45 minutes, and they should never take longer than an hour. (Some days you need to rest a bit longer, which adds time, as does doing abs.)

The usual reason why people's workouts pass into the 90+ minute range is that they don't pay attention to their rest times and chat with friends in between sets (leading to 5, 7, and even 10-minute rest times in between sets).

Long workouts are harmful in a couple of ways. First, it's hard to maintain mental and physical intensity for an hour and a half (especially when you're goofing off for 5 minutes in between sets). Second, when you exercise, your body produces hormones including testosterone, growth hormone, and cortisol. All three spike, and after about an hour of working out, your testosterone and growth hormone begin to fall, but your cortisol continues to rise. The more your cortisol rises, the more catabolic your body becomes. Continuing to train in this state causes symptoms of overtraining. In order to maintain anabolism, you want to end your training within about 60 minutes, and let your cortisol levels come down along with your testosterone and growth hormone levels.

Another benefit of shorter workouts is the simple fact that it's nice to not have to spend too much time in the gym every day. Pretty much anyone can figure out how to take an hour or so out of 3-5 days of each week to transform their body.

5-7
TRAIN EACH MUSCLE GROUP ONCE EVERY 5 – 7 DAYS

The amount of time you give a muscle group to rest before training it again plays a vital role in muscle growth (or lack thereof). Remember: You signal your muscles to grow by overloading them, but the growth itself occurs outside of the gym, when your body adapts the muscle to better deal with future overloads (by growing it bigger and stronger).

Recovery is what makes or breaks all of the above work to get you the body you want. If you don't allow your body to fully recover from a workout before you subject the same muscles to overload again, it doesn't matter how strictly you follow the rest of this training protocol—you will make minimal gains (and if you continue too long like this, you'll get weaker and flabbier, your energy levels will drop along with your appetite, and you'll lose all motivation for training).

Studies have shown that it takes the body 2-5 days to fully repair muscles after weight training. We experience this through the reduction of muscle soreness and inflammation, known as "delayed onset muscle soreness," or DOMs.

Now, our genetics, workout intensity and duration (how heavy you're training and how many sets you're doing), and overall fitness level determine how long our bodies need for recovery.

While some people will be fully recovered from the *Thinner Leaner Stronger* workouts in 3-4 days, I'm going to give you 5-7 days to ensure full recovery. It's not worth risking overtraining to try to sneak in an extra legs workout each week.

8-10
TAKE A WEEK OFF TRAINING EVERY 8 – 10 WEEKS

Lifting like this can be quite tough. It's heavy. It's intense. Your muscles will ache. Your joints will have to adapt.

Also, studies have shown that it takes 7-14 days for the central nervous system to fully recover from the stresses of weightlifting. As you'll be training 3-5 days per week, your CNS will get progressively overloaded, and will need a complete rest periodically.

Taking a week off training every couple of months is actually an important part of overall recuperation and recovery. After 8-10 weeks of training, your body needs a lull to fully recover, and you'll actually feel this physically (come week 8 or 9, don't be surprised if you feel low on energy, kind of weak, disinterested in training—all symptoms of overtraining coming on).

Don't worry that you'll get weaker or fatter on your week off. It won't happen. To the contrary, if you eat correctly during your week off, your body can actually go into a hyper-anabolic state, and you can come back noticeably stronger.

Another important point of your week off is that you don't want to do any strenuous physical activity during the week (no weightlifting, no strenuous cardio). You don't have to be a slug, but you don't want to give your body any unnecessary stresses to deal with.

Now, if after your first week off, you notice that you come back feeling lethargic and weaker, then I recommend that you try what I do: a "De-load Week."

For the longest time, I completely rested for one week every couple of months or so, but my body seemed to not like it. I rarely would come back stronger, whereas my friends would. What I do now works much better.

I come to the gym each day and instead of doing my normal workouts of heavy lifting, I do 6-9 light sets with 40-50% of my normal weight, and I never go to failure. I do 8-10 reps each set, which gives a bit of a pump, and nothing more. Remember that your CNS needs time to rebalance itself, so you don't want to put your body under any serious stress.

Studies have shown that increased blood flow (and nutrients) to the muscles helps improve recovery and protein synthesis, which is all I'm looking to accomplish.

For the first 6-9 months of being on this program, I recommend that you try weeks of complete rest. If you definitely don't like how your body feels after trying a few full rest weeks, or if you come back weaker, then try the "De-load Week." I think you'll like it.

CARDIO

A lot of people bash cardio simply because they don't like doing it. I know because I used to be one of them.

There are 3 primary ways that cardio can help you build (and retain) more muscle. They are as follows:

1. It improves muscle recovery by increasing blood flow to muscles.

2. It improves your body's metabolic responses to food, helping you minimize fat storage.

3. It keeps up your conditioning, making the transition from "bulking" to "cutting" easier on your body.

That said, *too much* cardio can negative affect your gains by reducing your caloric surplus too much, and by causing you to overtrain. If you just follow my recommendations, however, you shouldn't have any issues with this.

IS CARDIO BEST BEFORE OR AFTER LIFTING? NEITHER!

Doing cardio right before or after lifting can seriously hinder muscle and strength gains. Why?

Researchers from RMIT University worked with well-trained athletes in 2009 and found that "combining resistance exercise and cardio in the same session may disrupt genes for anabolism." In laymen's terms, they found that combining endurance and resistance training sends "mixed signals" to the muscles[26].

Cardio before the resistance training suppressed anabolic hormones such as IGF-1 and MGF, and cardio after resistance training increased muscle tissue breakdown.

Several other studies, such as those conducted by Children's National Medical Center[27], the Waikato Institute of Technology[28], and the University of Jyvaskyla (Finland)[29], came to same conclusions: training for both endurance and strength simultaneously impairs your gains on both fronts. Training purely for strength or purely for endurance in a workout is far superior.

Cardio before weightlifting also saps your energy and makes it much harder to train heavy, which in turn inhibits your muscle growth.

So, how do you do it right?

THE 3 COMMANDMENTS OF CARDIO

Whether you're doing cardio for the health benefits, because you like it, or to help with losing fat, here's how you prevent it from getting in the way of your muscle gains.

1. Do cardio 2-5 times per week.

Studies have shown that 3 cardio sessions per week is enough to improve cardiovascular function and muscle growth. Therefore, even if you're maintaining, I recommend that you do cardio at least 3 days per week.

Most woman find cardio necessary in order to get into the "super lean" category (15% and under) because you can only cut calories so much before you lose strength and muscle. I have to do cardio to get below 10%, for example, because I simply can't cut my calories any further without feeling miserable.

Some people, however, don't need to bother. They simply regulate their calories and get as lean as they want. This really is just a matter of genetics and individual physiology. You'll find out which category you fall into when you actually diet to lose weight, but you should plan on doing cardio 3-5 times per week to facilitate your fat loss.

2. Do high-intensity interval training (HIIT) cardio for 20-30 minutes per session.

Long, low-intensity cardio sessions tend to negatively impact muscle growth and burn relatively few calories, thus rendering them ineffective in helping with fat loss.

Studies such as those conducted by Laval University[30], East Tennessee State University[31], Baylor College of Medicine[32], and the University of New South Whales[33] have shown that shorter, high-intensity sessions, however, not only cause less muscle breakdown than low-intensity, steady-state cardio, but they burn more calories and stimulate more fat loss.

Therefore, I recommend doing HIIT for all cardio, and keeping your sessions 20-30 minutes long. Here's how it works:

- You start your workout with 2-3 minutes of low-intensity warm-up.

- You then go all-out, as fast as possible, for 30-60 seconds (if you're new to HIIT, 30-second intervels will be plenty, but you want to try to work toward being able to do 60-second intervals).

- You then slow it down to a low-intensity recovery period for the same period as your high-intensity interval. Again, if you're new to HIIT, you may need to extend this rest period to 1.5-2 times as long as your high-intensity interval. If you're still out of breath and your heart is racing, you're not ready to hit the high-intensity again.

- You repeat this cycle of all-out and recovery intervals for 20-30 minutes.

- You do a 2-3 minute cool-down at a low intensity.

You can apply the HIIT style to any type of cardio that you would normally do. You can head outside and walk and sprint, or you can hop on the elliptical trainer or recumbent bike to get it done.

3. Separate your weights and cardio sessions by several hours.

You already know why you need to separate your cardio and weight training, but unfortunately the studies didn't include a recommendation as to how much time you should put in between them.

I've tried many different intervals and found that a minimum of 2-3 hours seems to be best. Theoretically speaking, the longer you wait is probably better. I currently put about 14 hours in between my weights and cardio because I lift early in the morning and do cardio around 9:30 pm.

If there is no way that you can split up your cardio and weightlifting, I recommend doing your cardio after lifting (never before) and doing no more than 20-30 minutes of HIIT. This isn't an ideal setup, but it's not going to ruin your strength gains.

LIFTING WEIGHTS WHILE DIETING TO LOSE WEIGHT

Probably the worst training advice given to women who are trying to get lean is to train with light weights in order to get "really cut." This is 100% wrong. Lighter weights don't help burn more fat than heavier weights. They don't "really bring out definition." They don't make you toned. They're just a waste of time, really.

Training heavy is ESPECIALLY important when you're dieting to lose weight because that's how you're going to preserve your muscle—you're going to *force* your body to maintain its muscle by continuing to overload it.

If you really nail your diet and continue to train hard, don't be surprised if you actually gain some strength and muscle while losing fat. (If you have guy friends that lift weights, tell them this and they'll be jealous!)

THE BOTTOM LINE

These are the core fundamentals of *Thinner Leaner Stronger's* weight training program. Chances are that this is a new approach to lifting for you, and if that's the case, you should be excited.

Soon you're going to be enjoying steady, noticeable muscle growth (without getting bulky!) by doing relatively short, stimulating workouts that get the kind of results other women can only dream about.

19

MEET YOUR MAKERS: THE THREE LIFTS THAT BUILD GREAT BODIES

MOST PEOPLE TRAIN WITH IMPROPER form.

They'll stop their Bench Presses six inches or more above their chest and say that it's "better for their shoulders." They'll load up a bunch of plates and squat down a foot or two and stand back up, because they "don't want to stress their knees." They'll hunch their back when doing Deadlifts so they can "really go heavy," and heavily arch their lower back at the top to "really get a squeeze."

Well, not only does improper form stunt gains, it opens the door to injury. Heavy, half-reps on the Bench Press put unnecessary strain on your shoulders. Half-squats are, in fact, bad for your knees, while a full range of motion with manageable weights actually strengthens them. Hunched reps and over-arching of the back when deadlifting is a nasty injury just waiting to happen.

On the flip side, if you lift with strict attention to form and a full range of motion, you'll enjoy full development of your muscles, steady gains, and no unnecessary injuries or pains.

So, let's go over proper form for some of the key exercises that you will be doing as a part of this program.

THE SQUAT

Anyone that squats properly immediately gets my respect in the gym, regardless of the weight they're using.

Unfortunately, very, very few people actually do it right. The most common error is, of course, doing partial reps by not lowering the body until the hips drop lower than the knees. Shallow squats lead to all kinds of knee problems, especially when done with heavier weights, whereas proper squats actually strengthen the supporting muscles to the knees and prevent injury.

When performed correctly, the Squat is a safe, incredibly powerful exercise that you will come to love because of how beneficial it is to your entire body.

SQUAT SETUP

Always squat in a Power Rack or Squat Rack, with the safety bars/pins set six inches or so below the height of the bar at the bottom of the rep (which you'll learn about in a minute). Do this even if you have a spotter.

Position the bar on the rack so it cuts across the upper half of your chest. This might feel a bit low, but it's better to have it on the lower side than trying to tippy-toe the bar off the rack.

Face the bar so you can walk it out backward. Don't ever walk the bar out forward, as trying to re-rack it by walking backward is very dangerous.

Get under the bar and place your heels at about shoulder-width apart, with the toes pointed out at about 30-degree angles (your right foot at about 1 o'clock, and your left at about 11 o'clock, if that helps with the visual).

When you're ready to unrack the bar, bring your shoulder blades together, tighten your entire upper back, raise your chest up, and straighten your lower back. Put the bar below the bone at the top of your shoulder blades, solidly across your upper back muscles and rear deltoids.

Use a narrow grip because this helps you maintain upper-back tightness. Place your thumbs on top of the bar.

Here's a picture to help:

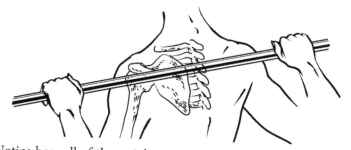

Notice how all of the weight is resting on her back, with none on her hands. This is important. The wide grip that many people use slackens the back muscles, which provide crucial support for the weight, and transfers the load to the spine. Don't follow their lead.

This position will probably feel a bit awkward at first, and you might need to stretch your shoulders to get your hands into the proper position. Whatever you do, do NOT put the bar on your neck!

If you really can't get the bar this low yet due to shoulder inflexibility, that's okay. Place it as close to this position as possible and as you continue to train, work on getting to this ideal position. As long as you don't feel it resting on your neck or feel your hands supporting the weight, you'll be fine.

SQUAT MOVEMENT

Once you've unracked the weight, take one or two steps back, and assume the proper squatting position as outlined above (heels shoulder-width apart, toes pointed out).

Pick a spot on the floor about six feet away, and stare at that for the entirety of the set. Don't look up at the ceiling as some people advise as this alone completely ruins form—it makes it almost impossible to reach the proper bottom position, it throws off proper hip movement and chest positioning, and it can cause a neck injury.

You're now ready to start the downward motion, which is accomplished by shifting the hips back and sitting the butt straight down while keeping the chest up, and the back straight and tight.

Many people have the tendency to want to transfer the load to the quads as the squat gets deep. One way to do this is to slide the knees forward, which can lead to weird pains and problems. A good rule of thumb is that any forward motion of the knees should occur in the first third or half of the descent, and the knees should go no further than just in front of the toes. Once the knees are out of the way and in place, the movement becomes a straight drop of the hips, followed by a straight lift of them.

The bottom of the squat is the point where your hips are back and slightly lower than your kneecaps (which causes your femurs to be a little lower than parallel with the ground), your knees are just a little forward of the toes and pointing in the same direction as your feet (out about a 30-degree angle, not in), and the back is as straight as possible and at an angle that places the bar over the middle of the foot.

I know that's a bit hard to visualize, so here's a simple diagram to help:

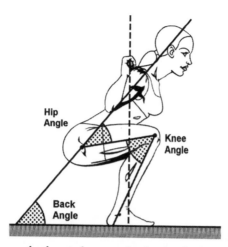

As you can see, the bar is low on the back, the back is completely flat and inclined at about a 45-degree angle, the hips are a little lower than the knees, the femurs are slightly past parallel, the feet are flat on the floor, and the knees are a little forward of the toes. This is the proper bottom of the Squat.

I recommend that you practice this with no bar to really get a feel for it. If you're having trouble getting your knees to point in line with your feet, you can, at the bottom, place your elbows against your knees and the palms of your hands together, and nudge your knees out.

If you need to place the bar a bit higher on your back due to shoulder stiffness, the angles change slightly. Here's another diagram to help:

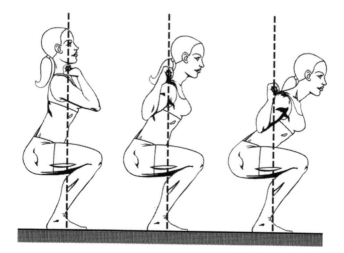

All the way to the left is the proper bottom position for the Front Squat. The middle is a high-bar Squat, and the far right is the low-bar Squat that I recommend you get comfortable doing.

Once you've reached the bottom, you drive your butt straight up—not forward—and bring your shoulders up at the same pace. To do this, you must maintain a back angle that keeps the weight over the middle of your foot. If your hips rise faster than your shoulders, you'll start tipping forward, which puts heavy strain on the neck and back.

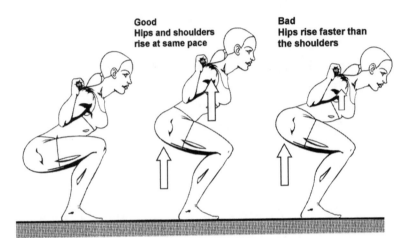

Good
Hips and shoulders
rise at same pace

Bad
Hips rise faster than
the shoulders

Don't think about anything but driving your hips straight up, and you'll do it correctly. Keep your chest up and your back straight—don't let it hunch.

SQUAT TIPS

Take a deep breath at the top of the first rep—when you're standing tall—and hold it, tightening your entire torso. Don't fully exhale during the set. You can completely hold your breath, or exhale slightly (maybe 10% of the air you're holding) on the way up for each rep, and then fill up with air again at the top.

Don't squat on a Smith Machine, as the fixed range of motion will prevent you from performing the exercise correctly and can hurt the knees.

If your back tends to round at the bottom, it's because your hamstrings are too tight. Stretch them every day (but not before lifting, as studies have shown that this saps strength[34] and does nothing to prevent the risk of injury[35]), and as they loosen, you'll find that you can keep your back straight for the entire lift.

Don't point your feet straight forward as this puts quite a lot of stress on the knees. As the stance widens, the body naturally wants the feet to be parallel with the thighs. By twisting the feet in, you put torque on the knees and, when loaded with weight and squatting deep, this can lead to injuries.

You can start your movement upward by creating a little "bounce" at the very bottom of the squat as your hamstrings, glutes, and groin muscles stretch to the limit of their natural ranges of motion. Don't pause at the bottom of the lift but instead use this slight bounce to initiate the drive upward.

If you're having trouble keeping your knees pointed out during the lift, you can take light (or no) weight and squat with your toes picked up off the ground, placing all the weight on your heels. By doing this, you will have no choice but to point your knees outward. Do this for a few reps, and then settle into the middle of your foot and do a few more reps, paying attention to the knees. Repeat this until you have it perfect.

Don't use a powerlifter's wide squatting stance. This type of stance does allow for more weight to be lifted, but it reduces the role of the quads.

Don't squat with a block under your heels, as this is done to compensate for a lack of hamstring flexibility. Instead, squat as described in this chapter and work on getting lower and lower, stretching your hamstrings. If you stick to it, you'll get there.

THE BENCH PRESS

Most women think of the Bench Press as the quintessential guy exercise. When guys want to judge each others' overall fitness, they usually ask, "How much do you bench?"

What you may not know, though, is that it's also a great exercise for women. It works not only the pectorals, which can give your chest a natural lift, it strengthens your shoulders, triceps, and back.

People's desire to bench a lot often leads to many mistakes, however: failing to bring the weight all the way down, over-arching the back, rolling the shoulders, flaring the elbows, and more. I see these things literally every day and will often say something, as improper form with heavy weight is how injuries occur.

So, how do you do the Bench Press properly?

BENCH PRESS SETUP

A strong Bench Press starts with a strong base. A strong base requires the right setup.

Squeeze your shoulder blades together before getting into position, and keep your back squeezed and down for the entire lift.

Your back should have a slight arch before and during the lift. The space created between your lower back and the bench should be just enough to snugly fit a fist, but not more.

Raise your chest as if you're going to show it to someone and keep it "up" for the entire lift.

If your grip is too narrow, you'll lose strength. If it's too wide, you'll reduce the range of motion and thus effectiveness of the exercise. Your grip width should be a few inches wider than shoulder-width (about 22-28 inches, depending on your build).

A common mistake is the "thumbless" grip, where you don't wrap your thumbs around the bar but place them next to your index fingers instead. While some people give various reasons for liking the thumbless grip, the reason to not use it is when you're going heavy, it's very easy to have the barbell slip out of your hands and crash down on your chest (just Google "thumbless grip bench press accident" if you don't believe me!).

Put the bar in the palm of your hand, not in your fingers, because this leads to wrist pains.

Grip the bar hard. Try to crush it like spaghetti. Believe it or not, this will give you a little boost in strength.

Your elbows should be pointing out from the body at about a 45-60-degree angle (between parallel and perpendicular to your torso). Keep your elbows "tucked" like this the entire time. Flaring them out puts undue stress on the shoulders.

Here's an image to help:

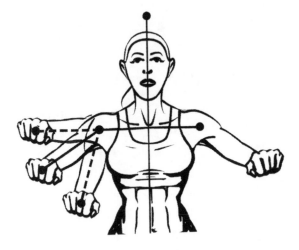

Plant your feet firmly on the floor with the weight on the heels, and space them widely apart. The upper part of your leg should be parallel to the floor, and the lower part should be perpendicular (forming a 90-degree angle), which improves strength and prevents heavy arching of the back.

Don't put your feet on the end of the bench—keep them on the floor. The knees-up position is less stable than the conventional position, and shouldn't be used with heavy weights.

BENCH PRESS MOVEMENT

The proper bench press form is a controlled movement of bringing the bar all the way down to the very bottom of your chest, followed by an explosive drive upward. The bar should move in a straight line up and down, not toward your face or belly button.

Here's an image to help:

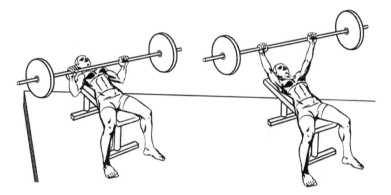

There is often debate over the point of whether you should bring the bar to your chest or not. Many fitness experts claim that you should lower the weight no further than the point where your upper arm is parallel to the floor, as doing this reduces the possibility of injury to the shoulders. This is nonsense.

Reducing the range of motion only reduces the effectiveness of the exercise, and Bench Press-related shoulder injuries are caused by improper technique, such as rolling the shoulders at the top and flaring the elbows out.

The possibility of injury will be greatly reduced (if not entirely eliminated) by maintaining perfect form, and a full range of motion will give you better muscle development in both your chest and shoulders.

BENCH PRESS TIPS

Unrack the bar by getting into position (pinching your shoulder blades, arching your back slightly, and pushing your chest up), locking your elbows out to move the bar off the hooks, and moving the bar into position with your elbows still locked. Don't try to bring the weight straight from the hooks to your chest. Don't drop your chest and loosen your shoulder blades when unracking, because it will make you shrug the bar off with your shoulders.

To help with lifting the bar straight up and down, look at the ceiling during the exercise and see the bar coming up, stopping in relation to a feature on the ceiling, and then going down. When you bring it back up, bring it up to the same spot in relation to the feature you've spotted on the ceiling. Don't watch the bar as it moves as you will inevitably vary its angle of descent and ascent.

Don't allow your chest to go flat while doing the press, and don't allow your shoulders to roll forward.

Use your legs to drive against the floor, which transfers force up through the hips and back and helps maintain proper form and increase strength.

Keep your butt on the bench at all times. If your butt is lifting, the weight is probably too heavy.

Don't bounce the bar off your chest. Lower it in a controlled manner keeping everything tight, let it touch your chest, and drive it up.

Don't smash the back of your head into the bench, as this can strain your neck. Your neck will naturally tighten while doing the exercise, but don't forcefully push it down.

When you're lowering the weight, think about the coming drive up. Visualize the explosive second half of the exercise the entire time, and you'll find it easier to control the descent of the weight, prevent bouncing, and even prepare your muscles for the imminent stress of raising the weight. (This technique is good for all exercises, by the way.)

Make sure to finish your last rep before trying to rack the weight. Many people make the mistake of moving the bar toward their face on the way up during their last rep, and this is dangerous (what if you miss the rep and it starts coming down?) and bad for the shoulders. Press the weight straight up as usual, lock your elbows out, and move the bar back to the rack until it hits the uprights, and then lower it to the hooks (don't go for the hooks first because you might miss them).

BENCH PRESS VARIATIONS

As a part of my program, you're going to do two variations of the Bench Press: the Close-Grip Bench Press, and the Incline Bench Press.

Incline Bench Press

The Incline Bench Press heavily involves the shoulders and upper part of the chest, and is a useful exercise to work into your routines.

When doing this exercise, the angle of incline in the bench should be 30-45 degrees. The basic setup and movement is just as you learned for the flat Bench Press, and the bar should pass by the chin and touch just below the collarbones. This will allow for a vertically straight bar path.

Close-Grip Bench Press

As you narrow your grip on the bar, the chest does less work, and the triceps do more. Thus, the Close-Grip Bench Press is a great exercise for targeting your triceps.

When doing a Close-Grip Bench Press, your grip should be slightly narrower than shoulder-width. The rest of the setup and movement is exactly as you just learned.

If your wrists hurt at the bottom of the lift, simply widen your grip by about the width of a finger and try again. If they still hurt, repeat until there's no pain.

You'll probably find that you fail much more suddenly on the Close-Grip Bench Press than the regular Bench Press. That's because the Close-Grip variation is relying mainly on the triceps, which are a smaller muscle group than the pectorals. Ensure your spotter knows this, and if you don't have a spotter, don't try for that next rep if you don't think you can make it.

THE DEADLIFT

Like the Squat, the Deadlift is one of the toughest and most rewarding lifts you can do. When you see someone deadlifting big weight with perfect form, you're witnessing a rare, admirable feat.

This program will have you deadlift regularly, and there are many ways to mess this lift up, so I want to take a few pages to fully describe proper form.

DEADLIFT SETUP AND MOVEMENT

Always start with the bar on the floor—not on the safety pins or on the rack.

Your stance should be a bit narrower than shoulder-width, and your toes should be pointed slightly out. You should stand with the bar above the middle of your feet (the top of your instep).

Bend at your waist and grip the bar by placing it into the middle of your palms, not in your fingers. Both palms should be facing in to build grip strength. The other grip option is the "alternate" method where one palm faces in (usually the non-dominant hand) and the other faces out, which can allow for heavier weight to be lifted, but can also be uncomfortable.

Your arms should be just outside your legs, leaving enough room for your thumbs to clear your thighs.

Bend through your knees until your shins touch the bar, and then lift your chest until your back is in a neutral position and tight. Don't over-arch your back, and don't squeeze your shoulder blades together like with the Squat. Just push your chest up and your shoulders and back down. Your arms should be completely straight and locked.

Here's what this position looks like:

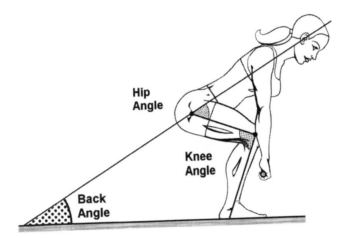

You're now ready to pull.

Take a deep breath, look forward, and start the upward movement by engaging the quads to begin the straightening of the knees. This will pull the bar up your shins, and once the weight is off the ground, join your hips into the upward movement and keep your back neutral and tight the whole way up. You should try to keep the bar on as vertically straight of a path as possible (absolute isn't attainable, but there should be little lateral movement of the bar as you lift it up).

The bar should move up your shins, and roll over your knees and thighs. At the top, your chest should be out and your shoulders down. Don't lean back, shrug the weight, or roll your shoulders up and back.

Here's how the entire first half of the lift looks:

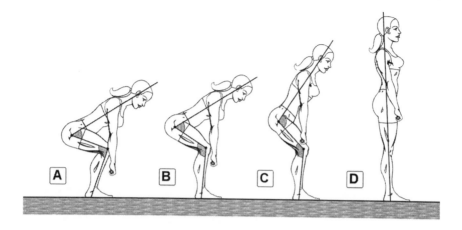

The next half of the movement is lowering the weight back down to the floor in a controlled manner (yes, it must go all the way back to the floor!). This is simply a mirror image of what you did to come up.

You begin to lower the bar by pushing your hips back first, letting the bar descend in a straight line until it reaches your knees. At that point, you bend your knees and lower it down your shins. The back stays locked in its tight, neutral position the entire time.

Here's how it looks:

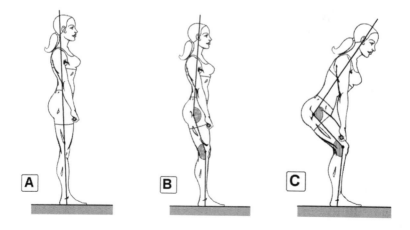

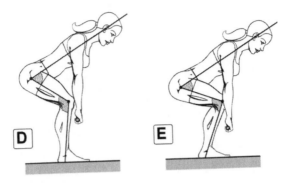

DEADLIFT TIPS

Don't start with your hips too low. Remember that the Deadlift starting position is not the same as the Squat bottom position. The Deadlift requires that your hips be higher than the bottom of the Squat.

When you're lowering the weight, if you break your knees too early, you'll hit them with the bar. To avoid this, begin your descent by pushing your hips back first and don't bend your knees until the bar reaches your knees.

If you start the upward motion with bent elbows, you'll end up putting unnecessary strain on your biceps. Keep your elbows straight for the entire lift.

Deadlifting in shoes that have air cushions or gel filling is a bad idea. It compromises stability, causes power loss, and interferes with proper form. Get shoes with flat, hard soles like Chuck Taylors.

Wear long pants and long socks on the day that you'll be deadlifting to prevent shin scraping. Shin scraping can be caused by poor form, but can also be unavoidable depending on the length of the limbs and body type.

Too wide of a stance or grip will make the exercise awkward. The Deadlift stance is narrower than the Squat stance, and the Deadlift requires that the hands be just outside the legs.

Don't strain to look up while deadlifting. Keep your head in a neutral position and in line with your spine.

If you start the upward lift with your hips too high, you'll turn the Deadlift into a Stiff-Legged Deadlift, which is more stressful on the lower back and hamstrings. Make sure that you get your hips low enough in the starting position (but not too low!).

Explode the bar up from the floor as fast as you can. Apply as much force as quickly as possible and you'll be able to move more weight.

Try to crush the bar with your grip. If your knuckles aren't white, you're not squeezing hard enough.

DEADLIFT VARIATIONS

Romanian Deadlift

The "RDL," as it's often called, was started by a Romanian powerlifter named Nicu Vlad, who would perform outrageous feats of strength like front squatting 700 lbs while only weighing 220 lbs.

The RDL is a variation of the Deadlift that targets the glutes and hamstrings, and minimizes the involvement of the quads and hip muscles.

The RDL starts with the weight on safety pins or the lower portion of the rack. The same stance and grip is used as the Deadlift, and the weight is walked back a step or two. In the start position, the knees are locked, the chest is up, the back is straight and tight, and the eyes are focused on a point on the floor about ten feet away.

When the movement is begun, the knees are unlocked just enough to put some tension on the quads, and the back is slightly arched. The bar is started down the thigh in a straight line by pushing the hips back, and the torso leans forward to keep the shoulders directly over the bar. As the bar approaches the knees, move them back, out of the way, and drop the bar past the knees, moving it along the shins. Go as low as you can without breaking the extension of your back.

Resist the temptation to relax the tension in the knees at the bottom by flexing them, as this transfers the load from the hamstrings to the quads.

Once you've achieved a good stretch in your hamstrings and your back is ready to unlock, start back up. On the way up, keep your chest and back tight and locked into position, and move the bar along your legs.

Because of the increasing angle of the torso, you probably won't be able to go much further than a few inches past your knees, and that's okay. In fact, if the weight is touching the floor, you're doing it wrong (you're bending your knees).

Make sure to hold your back rigid for the entire lift. Don't let the chest sag or the lower back loosen.

THE REST OF THE EXERCISES YOU'LL BE DOING

You'll be doing more exercises than those I've covered thus far, of course, but I wanted to give the Squat, Bench Press, and Deadlift special attention as they are essential for building a great body, but particularly problematic if performed incorrectly.

For the rest of the exercises you're going to be doing in the program, I could write another several pages, but I think it will be better if you simply watch videos as there just aren't very many technical points to doing them correctly.

The best videos that I've found is offered by <u>bodybuilding.com</u>, which you can find at <u>www.bodybuilding.com/exercises</u>. Their videos won't teach you everything you now know about the core barbell exercises, but they are fine for simpler movements like the Dumbbell Curl, Front Lat Pull Down, Leg Press, and so forth. You can also download the bonus report, which has links to all the videos you'll need.

Make sure to watch the videos for each exercise before you do them for the first time.

IS A SPOTTER NECSSARY?

Although having a spotter isn't entirely necessary as you should only be handling weight that you can do clean, unassisted reps with, it does help for a couple of reasons.

First, it allows you to get that one extra rep that you might not want to try otherwise, especially with exercises like Bench Press and Squats.

Second, there's a strange strength benefit to having someone standing there to assist you, even if they do nothing more than put their hands, or even fingers, under the bar. I know it sounds like a myth, but you'll experience it—you'll be struggling on your last rep, your partner will just put his or her fingers under the bar, and suddenly you'll push it up.

If you don't have someone to work out with, I recommend that you ask someone to give you a spot when necessary. It'll help.

When you're spotting another, the proper way to do it is like this:

1. Help them with the lift off if necessary (such as with the Close-Grip Bench Press and Military Press).

2. Let them do the reps without any assistance from you.

3. If they get bogged down on a rep, first just put your hands in place to help.

4. If they're still stuck, take maybe 10% of the load off.

5. If they're still stuck, take another 10-15% of the load off.

6. If they're still stuck, they're toast and just take as much of the load

off as you can.

I don't want to make this sound complicated, but a good spotter is there for safety reasons only, and if you're moving the weight up, she doesn't touch it. She only ends the set when totally necessary.

While the technique of spotting is self-explanatory in most cases, I'd like to mention here the proper way to spot someone who's squatting. The key is to the spot the bar, not the person. Don't hook your arms under the lifter's armpits as the purpose of spotting is to lift weight off, and spotting the person's body isn't the safest way to do this.

20

YOUR *THINNER LEANER STRONGER* WORKOUT PLAN

NOW THAT YOU KNOW EXACTLY how to eat and train for maximum results, all you need to get started is an exact training plan to follow. Well, let's get to it.

DON'T FORGET THE FORMULA

First and foremost, you must always apply what you learned in the *Thinner Leaner Stronger* training formula. How you train is just as important as what exercises you do. If you followed the workouts given in this chapter but violated the formula, you'd make less-than-optimum gains. On the flip side, if you followed the formula but did the wrong exercises, you'd also make less-than-optimum gains.

When you combine consistent application of the formula with the proper exercises, you can completely transform your physique. And that's what this training plan is going to give you.

WARMING UP

Before you do your first "heavy" set when weight training, you want to warm up the muscle group that you'll be working.

The purpose of the warm-up is to infuse enough blood into the muscle and connective tissues so that they can be maximally recruited to handle the heavy sets.

The warm-up should not fatigue your muscles. It should simply fill them with blood and prepare the tendons and ligaments for the stress of the heavier sets.

It's very easy to do.

FIRST WARM-UP SET

For your fist warm-up set, you do 12 reps with about 50% of your "heavy" weight (weight that only allows for 8-10 reps), and then you rest for 1 minute. Don't rush this set, but don't take it too slowly either. It will feel very light and easy.

So, if you did 3 sets of 9 with 100 lbs on your Squats last week, you would start your warm-up at 50 lbs and do 12 reps, followed by 1 minute of rest.

SECOND WARM-UP SET

For your second warm-up set, you use the same weight as the first and do 10 reps this time at a little faster pace. Then rest for 1 minute.

THIRD WARM-UP SET

Your third set is 6 reps with about 70% of your heavy weight, and it should be done at a moderate pace. It should still feel light and easy. This set and the following one are to acclimate your muscles to the heavy weights that are about to come. Once again, you follow this with a 1-minute rest.

FOURTH, FIFTH, AND SIXTH SETS:

These are your muscle-building, or "working," sets for the exercise.

MOVING ON TO THE NEXT EXERCISE:

Let's say you now are going to do Lunges. Should you do a whole other warm-up routine? The answer is no. Your muscles are completely warmed up and able to handle heavy weight, so why would you bother?

The only exception to this is the rare case of moving on to an exercise that involves muscles that would not have been warmed up, such as going from Lat Pulldowns to Deadlifts. If you start your back routine on the Lat Pulldown machine and warm up there, you'd be fine going straight into exercises like Barbell or Dumbbell Rows, Low Rows, V-Bar Pulldowns, Weighted Pull-Ups, and so on, but since Deadlifts put considerable stress on your lower back and hamstrings, you should do a few warm-up sets to prevent straining these muscles.

YOUR FIRST *THINNER LEANER STRONGER* TRAINING ROUTINE

This routine calls for five days of weightlifting, as much cardio as you'd like to do based on what your goals and what you now know, and two days of rest from the weights, and one day of complete rest (no exercise whatsoever).

If you can only train three or four days per week, I have a program for you, too, which I'll share at the end of this chapter. If there's any way that you can make the time to lift five days per week, however, do it. You'll make the most gains that way.

For example, here's what I do:

Mon – Fri: Lift

Sat: Complete rest

Sun – Tues/Weds: Cardio

This is easy and works for most, but you could also do something like the following:

Day 1: Lift & cardio

Day 2: Lift

Day 3: Cardio

Day 4: Lift & cardio

Day 5: Lift & cardio

Day 6: Rest

Day 7: Lift

You should do the following exercises each week for the first two months. As to what you should do after the first two months, I highly recommend that you download the free bonus report at the end of this book, because in it I fully lay out your first year in terms of training, dieting, and supplementing.

You should do the exercises in the order given. Start with the first exercise and do your warm-up sets, followed by your three heavy sets (with the proper rest in between each, of course). Then move on to the next exercise on the list, and so forth.

If you've never lifted heavy weights before or performed the exercises called for, your first week might feel a bit awkward as you get used to both the movements and weight ranges. Use your warm-up sets to get acquainted with the exercises, and feel free to work in the 10-12 or even 12-15 rep range for this first week to get a good feel for everything. Then, in week two, move into the 8-10 range.

In case you're not familiar with some or all of the exercises I give in this chapter, I just want to remind you that bodybuilding.com offers a great collection of videos, which you can find at www.bodybuilding.com/exercises. You can also find links to videos of every exercise for your first year of training in the bonus report.

I think this is a much better way to learn the exercises than looking at a few photos for each like what most books give you. So head on over to check the exercises out before you do them.

If you're new to lifting and you do the following exercises, applying the formula, training hard, and also eating correctly, you can expect to lose at least 10-15 pounds in your first two months (if weight loss is your goal), or gain a few pounds of muscle, which will make quite a difference in how your body looks.

DAY 1: Chest and Abs

Flat Bench Press – Warm-up sets and then 3 working sets (8-10 reps per set)

Incline Bench Press – 3 working sets (8-10 reps per set)

Incline Dumbbell Bench Press – 3 working sets (8-10 reps pre set)

Dips (Chest Variation) – 3 working sets to failure (use the assistance machine if necessary)

Cable Crunch – 3 sets (enough weight to allow 15-20 reps per set)

Captain's Chair Leg Raise – 3 sets (no weight, as many as you can do)

Air Bicycles (no weight, as many as you can do) – 3 sets

The Bench Press is one of the most effective chest-building exercises you can do, and by doing flat and incline presses, you'll be working each part of your chest. Dips are also one of my favorites because you can get a great stretch and hit your chest on an angle that weights just can't duplicate.

The most effective ab routine I've been able to come up with over the years relies on the three exercises given above. It's nothing fancy, but it will rock your core. What I do is, after a set of chest, go immediately to Cable Crunches. Once I've done that, I immediately do Leg Raises to failure, followed by Air Bicycles (also called "Air Bikes") to failure. I then rest 1-2 minutes and get back to chest. Three of these "supersets" and your abs will be crying for mercy. If you can work up to 5-6 full circiuts, you're a superstar.

DAY 2: Back

Barbell Deadlift – Warm-up sets and then 3 working sets

Barbell Row – 3 working sets

One-Arm Dumbbell Row – 3 working sets

Close-Grip Lat Pulldown – 3 working sets

All of these exercises are great overall back builders, and this combination will work your entire back.

If you have lower-back issues, skip the Deadlifts. At the end of this chapter, I provide other great exercises for each body part, so substitute in another "approved" exercise for the Deadlifts.

DAY 3: Shoulders

Seated Barbell Military Press – Warm-up sets and then 3 working sets

Barbell Upright Row – 3 working sets

Side Lateral Raise – 3 working sets

Bent-Over Rear Delt Raise – 3 working sets

The shoulder is a muscle (deltoid) that's comprised of 3 "heads": the anterior (front), lateral (side), and posterior (back). If you want full, round shoulders, you need to work each head, and these 3 exercises ensure that you fully work the entire muscle group.

DAY 4: Legs

Barbell Squat – Warm-up sets and then 3 working sets

Leg Press – 3 working sets

Barbell Lunge – 3 working sets

Romanian Deadlift – 3 working sets

Nothing beats Squats, Lunges, and Romanian Deadlifts for building toned, sexy legs and round, perky butts. You will get a ton of mileage from this workout.

If you have lower-back issues, skip the RDLs and substitute another "approved" exercise for them.

DAY 5: Arms

Alternating Dumbbell Curl – Warm-up sets and then 3 working sets

Triceps Pushdown – Warm-up sets and then 3 working sets

Barbell Curl – 3 working sets

Seated Triceps Press – working 3 sets

These four arm exercises are some of the best you can do. Hit these hard and your arms will look great!

WANT MORE WORKOUT ROUTINES?

In talking with readers, some like to take what they've learned in this book and formulate their own plans, while others would like a little help with coming up with more routines.

Therefore, I decided to create a full year's worth of training routines, and I've included it in the free bonus report that you'll find at the end of this book. Check it out when you get there!

IF YOU CAN ONLY TRAIN 3 OR 4 DAYS PER WEEK

If there's no way for you to lift five days per week, don't despair. While three days of training per week won't be as effective as five, you can still make great gains.

The following three-day program has worked best for me:

Day 1: Chest (warm up and 12 working sets) & tris (6 working sets, no warm-up needed)

Day 2: Back (warm up and 12 working sets) & bis (6 working sets, no warm-up needed)

Day 3: Legs (warm up and 12 working sets) & shoulders (warm up and 12 working sets)

You do the same workouts given earlier in this chapter. You just have to double them up each day. To prevent the workouts from taking forever, I recommend that you do the following:

Set 1 for muscle A and then rest 60 seconds

Set 1 for muscle B and then rest 60 seconds

Set 2 for muscle A and then rest 60 seconds

Set 2 for muscle B and then rest 60 seconds

And so forth. If you stick to that, they're tough workouts, but you can wrap them all up in an hour or so.

You can do abs on 1-2 of your off days so your workouts don't take too long.

If you can only train four days per week, here's what I recommend:

Day 1: Chest (warm up and 12 working sets) & tris (6 working sets, no warm-up needed)

Day 2: Back (warm up and 12 working sets) & bis (6 working sets, no warm-up needed)

Day 3: Shoulders (warm up and 12 working sets) & abs

Day 4: Legs (warm up and 12 working sets)

I would rather double up on chest and back days than doing a legs and shoulders day, because the latter is just grueling.

If you want to do one extra day of abs, do it on day 6.

YOUR FIRST FEW WEEKS

For the first 2-3 weeks, you'll probably find many exercises a bit awkward. You'll be discovering your weight ranges, and you'll probably experience various aches and stiffness. All of this is normal and just part of the game. It shouldn't take long before you're comfortable with each exercise and your weight for each, however, and the aches will subside.

Sharp pains while lifting, however, mean that something is wrong. Don't try to muscle through a sharp pain. Instead, drop the weight and check your form. If your form is fine, stop the exercise and do another.

Stay away from the exercise that was giving you pain for a few weeks and strengthen the area with an exercise that doesn't hurt. Then try the original again and see if it still bothers you. If it still does, don't do it.

If you're having any serious pains, see a doctor as it might be an indicator of something else.

CHANGING IT UP

While the idea of "muscle confusion" is stupid and unfounded, it is true that your body can respond favorably to doing new exercises after doing the same routine for a bit. Thus, it's good to change your routine every couple of months.

What I like to do is change out an exercise or two from each workout every 8-10 weeks (after my rest or De-load Week). I'll then do that new routine for the next 8-10 weeks, take a week off, change up the exercises, and keep the pattern going.

The key is that you substitute the *right* exercises, however, so below I've listed the exercises that you can choose from. I recommend only these because they are the most effective exercises that you can do for each muscle group.

CHEST

Dumbbell Press (flat, incline)

Barbell Bench Press (flat, incline)

Push-Up

Dip

I usually rotate between dumbbell-centric and barbell-centric routines. For example, I'll do a routine of Incline Dumbbell Presses, Flat Dumbbell Press, and Dips for 2-3 months, and then switch to a routine of Flat Bench Press, Incline Bench Press, and Flat Dumbbell Press for the next 2-3 months.

I recommend that you always do at least one incline press in your chest workout, as this is the toughest type of chest exercise you can do.

Finally, I've done every chest routine you can imagine and I've intentionally left off certain exercises that people often do.

One example is the decline variation of presses, which are just not as effective as the flat and incline variations because they shorten the length of the rep (meaning less work is done by the muscle group). The argument for doing decline presses is that they work the lower chest, but the Dip is a far superior movement for this purpose, while also involving more overall muscles, more balance and coordination, and more nervous system stimulation.

I've also left out isolation exercises such as flyes and machine presses because they don't build muscle as effectively as the compound movements I've recommended.

BACK

Barbell Deadlift

Pull-Up

Chin-Up

One-Arm Dumbbell Row

T-Bar Row

Bent-Over Barbell Row

Front Lat Pulldown

Close-Grip Pulldown

Seated Cable Row (wide- and close-grip)

I highly recommend always keeping the Deadlift in your routine. You just can't beat it for all-around back development and strength. If you're careful to always keep proper form and not rush to handle more weight than you can properly lift, you shouldn't run into any of the lower-back or knee-related issues that people sometimes complain about.

So, most of your back workouts will start with Deadlifts. For your other two exercises, I recommend choosing a close-grip exercise for targeting the middle of your back, and a wide-gripped exercise for targeting your lats. The Pull-Up, T-Bar Row, and Bent-Over Barbell Row are especially effective choices as they work the entire back (middle-back and lats, and for the latter two, the lower-back as well).

A few workouts I really enjoy are Barbell Deadlift, T-Bar Row, and One-Arm Dumbbell Row; Barbell Deadlift, Bent-Over Barbell Row, Close-Grip Pulldown; and Barbell Deadlift, Front Lat Pulldown, Pull-Up.

SHOULDERS

Seated Barbell Military Press

Seated Dumbbell Press

Arnold Dumbbell Press

Dumbbell Front Raise

Barbell Upright Row

Side Lateral Raise

Bent-Over Rear Delt Raise

Seated Rear Delt Raise

I like to keep my shoulder workouts simple: one exercise for each head, always starting with an overhead press. My favorite overall exercise is the Seated Barbell Military Press, because it just blasts the anterior (front) head of the shoulder.

The Dumbbell Front Raise is a good exercise, but don't do this in place of the Military or Dumbbell Press as it simply doesn't build mass like those two do. If you're particularly weak on your press exercises, the Front Raise can be very helpful in strengthening many of the small, supporting muscles required for the tougher lifts, and it can be added to the end of your normal workout (making it 12 working sets). I also find that a rep range of 8-10 reps works best for this exercise.

I only have a few shoulder routines that I rotate through: Seated Barbell Military Press, Side Lateral Raise, Bent-Over Rear Delt Raise; Seated Barbell Military Press, Dumbbell Front Raise, Side Lateral Raise, Seated Rear Delt Raise; and Seated Dumbbell (or Arnold) Press, Side Lateral Raise, Seated Rear Delt Raise.

LEGS

Barbell Squat

Hack Squat

Front Squat

Barbell Lunge

Dumbbell Lunge

Leg Press

Romanian Deadlift

Leg Extension

Leg Curl

Working legs is very, very simple. Rule #1: Always do squats. Rule #2: Always do squats. Rule #3: You get the point.

My leg workouts always begin with Barbell Squats. From there, I like to do Hack Squats or the Leg Press, followed by a hamstring-centric exercise like the RDL or Leg Curl.

This is all it takes to build sexy, strong legs.

ARMS (BICEP):

Barbell Curl

Straight Bar Curl

E-Z Bar Curl

Dumbbell Curl

Hammer Curl

These exercises are all you need for the bicep. You can start with a bar curl or a dumbbell curl, and then do the opposite next. The Barbell Curl and Straight Bar Curl are widely considered the best overall muscle builders for the bicep, and I agree.

ARMS (TRICEPS):

Close-Grip Bench Press

Seated Triceps Press

Triceps Pushdown

Lying Triceps Extension

Dip

My favorite triceps exercises are the Close-Grip Bench Press and Seated Triceps Press. I do rotate through each of the exercises given above, however. My favorite pairings are Seated Triceps Press and Close-Grip Bench Press; Weighted Dip and Triceps Pushdown; and Close-Grip Bench Press and Weighted Dip.

ABS

Cable Crunch

Captain's Chair Leg Raise

Air Bicycles

Ab Roller

Decline Crunch

Hanging Leg Raise

Flat Bench Lying Leg Raise

As you know, the "secret" to having a great stomach is being lean, but it does take abs work to get the lines and definition that most women want. There are a million different exercises that people and magazines recommend for abs, but I've narrowed them down to the handful given above in terms of overall effectiveness.

When building your own abs routines, I recommend starting with a weighted exercise (you can add weight to leg raise exercises by snatching a dumbbell in between your feet, and while some people add weight to the Decline Crunch by holding a plate or dumbbell, I find this pretty awkward). You then follow it with two unweighted exercises done to failure.

My routine is pretty static here. I do the Cable Crunch, Captain's Chair Leg Raise, and then either Air Bicycles to burnout, or the Ab Roller to burnout.

THE BOTTOM LINE

Pretty simple, isn't it? Start with the first routine I gave you in this chapter and follow it for your first two months on the program.

Once you've completed your first two months and taken your rest week, it's time to switch out some exercises and build your strength on those for the next two months. After a year or so of doing this, you'll have a really good feel for your body and what it responds to best.

Once again, I recommend that you check out the bonus report at the end of this book as you can see how I would build your first year of training to maximize your gains.

21

THE NO-BS GUIDE TO
SUPPLEMENTS

Advanced time release formula guaranteed to feed your muscle for up to 8 hours!

Kick your metabolism into overdrive and burn fat 24 hours per day, 7 days per week!

Assault estrogen receptors in your body and completely block muscle-killing hormones!

THE SHELVES OF YOUR LOCAL GNC are packed with all kinds of magical wonder drugs claiming to deliver results that only steroids can achieve.

This includes pre-workout supplements, intra-workout supplements, post-workout supplements, fat loss supplements, test boosters, HGH boosters, nitric oxide supplements, anti-estrogens, aromatase inhibitors, and the list goes on and on.

If you believe half of the hype you read in supplement advertisements or on their labels, well, it would probably take a while before you realize the simple truth of the matter, which is…

Most everything you see in the world of workout supplements is utterly worthless.

Yup…a complete waste of money. Not all. But most.

How can I say that so confidently? I've not only tried every type of supplement you can imagine, but I've studied the science and only follow what has been objectively proven—not subjective testimony, shady "independent studies," or fancy marketing pitches.

You see, the supplement companies are cashing in BIG on a little trick that your mind can play on you known as the *placebo effect*. This is the scientifically proven fact that your simple belief in the effectiveness of a medicine or supplement can make it work. People have overcome every form of illness you can imagine, mental and physical, by taking substances which they *believed* to have therapeutic value, but which actually didn't. I'm talking about things like curing cancer and diabetes, eliminating depression and anxiety, and lowering blood pressure and cholesterol levels by taking medically worthless substances that the people *believed* were treatments for their problems.

Many guys *believe* that the shiny new bottle of "muscle-maximizing" pills will work, and then they sometimes actually do "feel them working" even though, it comes out later, the ingredients have never been scientifically proven to do anything the company claims. Or, it's revealed that the scientific trials they tout in their ads were fraudulent.

Many women fall into the same trap with fat-loss supplements that promise to magically get your body to burn only fat for its energy or drastically increase your metabolism so you become a fat-burning machine.

That said, there are a handful of supplements that actually are worth buying and using. They aren't the sexy fat burning crap pushed in the magazines, but they are scientifically proven to help you build muscle, lose fat, and stay healthy.

So, let's go through the common types of supplements out there and look at what you should and shouldn't spend your hard-earned cash on. And in the bonus report offered at the end of this book, and on my website (www.muscleforlife.com), you'll find my exact product recommendations (brands and products themselves).

PROTEIN SUPPLEMENTS

Protein is the nutrient most responsible for muscle growth and repair. Using protein supplements such as whey, egg, and casein powders (your three best options) isn't *necessary*, but it is *convenient*.

Unless you are in the lucky position of being able to have whole food meals ready 4-6 times per day, you're going to need to use protein supplements.

Whey protein is a staple in most athletes' diets for a good reason: it's digested quickly, absorbed efficiently, and easy on the taste buds.

Prices are all over the place, however, ranging from less than $10 per pound, to over $20 per pound, and marketing claims used to justify various price points range from sensible to ludicrous.

So what gives? Let's lift the veil of mystery on whey so you can make an informed choice, and get the right product for the right price.

Whey is a byproduct of cheese production. It's a relatively clear liquid left over after milk has been curdled and strained, and it used to be disposed of as waste. It was later discovered that it contains an impressive array of complete proteins necessary for protein synthesis and hypertrophy, and thus, the whey protein supplement was born.

But why is whey so big in the health and fitness world? Does it warrant all the attention?

Well, whey is especially popular with athletes and bodybuilders because of its amino profile, which is rich in leucine[36], an essential amino acid that plays a key role in initiating protein synthesis[37]. Research has also shown that whey helps the body regulate blood glucose levels after a meal[38].

Whey is particularly effective when eaten after training, due to its rapid digestion and abundance of leucine. Simply put, the faster protein is digested and the more leucine it has, the more muscle growth it stimulates[39], and research has proven that whey is a highly effective form of post-workout protein[40].

So yes, there's a good reason why most protein supplements sold are whey. But not all whey products are equal.

The three forms of whey protein sold are whey concentrate, isolate, and hydrolysate.

Whey concentrate is the least processed form and cheapest to manufacture, and it contains some fat and lactose. Whey concentrates range from 35-80% protein by weight[41], depending on quality.

Whey isolate is a form of whey protein processed to remove the fat and lactose. Isolates are 90%+ protein by weight[41]. As they're more expensive to manufacture than whey concentrate, they're more expensive for consumers too.

Whey hydrolysate is a predigested form of whey protein that's very easily absorbed by the body and free of allergenic substances found in milk products[42]. Research also indicates that the hydrolysis process improves solubility and digestibility[42]. Whey hydrolysate is the most expensive of the three options.

So which should you buy? Well, when choosing a whey, you have a few things to consider.

While isolates and hydrolysates are pushed as superior to concentrates due to purity and higher protein concentrations per scoop, there's insufficient evidence to support claims that they are superior to concentrates when used as a part of a mixed diet.

That said, choosing the cheapest whey you can find, which will always be a concentrate, isn't a good idea, either. A quality whey concentrate is somewhere around 80% protein by weight, but inferior concentrates can have as little as 30% protein by weight.

What else is in there, then?

Unfortunately we can only wonder, as adulteration (the addition of fillers like maltodextrin and flour) is startlingly rampant in this industry[43].

In many cases, you'll get what you pay for--if the product costs a lot less than the going rate for whey, it's probably because it's made with inferior ingredients.

High prices aren't always indicative of high-quality, though. Disreputable supplement companies also pull other tricks, such as starting with a low-quality concentrate, adding small amounts of isolate and hydrolysate to create a "blend," and then calling attention to the isolate and hydrolysate in their marketing and packaging.

To protect yourself as a consumer, always check ingredient lists and serving sizes and amounts of protein per serving before buying protein powder.

Specifically, you're going to want to look at the order in which the ingredients are listed (ingredients are listed in descending order according to predominance by weight), and the amount of protein per scoop relative to the scoop size.

For instance...

- If a product has maltodextrin (a filler), or any other ingredient, listed before the protein powder, don't buy it (that means there's more maltodextrin, creatine, or other fillers in it than protein powder).

- If a scoop is 40 grams but there is only 22 grams of protein per serving, don't buy it unless you know that the other 18 grams are made up of stuff you want (weight gainers have quite a few carbs per scoop, for instance).

A high-quality whey protein is easy to spot: whey concentrate, isolate, or hydrolysate listed as the first ingredients, and a scoop size relatively close to the amount of actual protein per scoop (it'll never match because there is at least sweetener and flavoring along with the protein powder in every serving).

Fortunately, there isn't as much to worry about with casein and egg supplements. Stick with a casein that uses micellar casein (the highest quality available), and most egg products are comparable, but I prefer one company specifically, which you'll find in the bonus report.

BCAAS

Branched Chain Amino Acids (BCAAs) are the three "building blocks" of your body: leucine, isoleucine, and valine. They make up about 35% of your muscle mass and must be present in the body for muscle growth and repair to occur.

While that description might lead you to assume that yes, you absolutely should be buying BCAA supplements…not so fast. Most whole food proteins are made up of about 15% BCAAs, and most protein supplements have BCAAs added, so when you're eating enough protein, especially if you're using protein supplements with BCAAs added, you're getting enough BCAAs to meet your body's demands[44].

I only recommend buying BCAAs under two circumstances:

1. When you're doing an abnormally high amount of muscularly strenuous activity each week, which puts incredibly high amino acid demands on the body (e.g., lifting weights five times per week and playing sports three days per week for a couple of hours each day).

2. When you're training in a fasted state, which is a state wherein you haven't eaten in 3+ hours and your insulin levels are low. Fasted training is useful for accelerating fat loss and for targeting stubborn fat in particular, but is also kind of an "advanced" topic. If you want to learn more about it, head over to my website (www. muscleforlife.com) and search for "stubborn fat."

PRE-WORKOUT DRINK

Advertisements for popular pre-workout products are some of the most exaggerated in the industry. Take 20 grams of powder and you'll experience "highly explosive energy," "maximum anabolic activation," and "extreme training endurance," they say. And they have pictures of monstrous bodybuilders that look like they're about to die of a heart attack to back it up.

What gives, though? Are these products actually worth it, or are you better off popping a couple caffeine pills or drinking an espresso instead?

Pre-workout products are notorious for a few deceitful practices:

- Including ineffective ingredients to make long, impressive nutrition labels, and using (and often mis-interpreting) cherry-picked, flawed, or biased studies to justify their use.

- Under-dosing key ingredients and hiding it behind the "proprietary blend" labeling loophole that allows companies to not disclose the actual composition of each part of the blend[45].

- Using chemical names of everyday compounds to mislead you into thinking the products have special ingredients. For instance, epigallo-3-catechin-3-O-b-gallate is just green tea extract, and 1,3,7-trimethylxanthine is just caffeine.

Why do these things?

Because it's *extremely profitable.*

You see, here's the game: When Shady Supplements, Inc. is looking to create a pre-workout product, they believe two things are key for sales: 1) being able to list ingredients on the label that have been clinically proven as safe and effective, so marketing claims can be defended, and 2) being able to list a bunch of other junk that sounds impressive, but which has no science to back it up, intended to give you the impression that you're getting a lot for your money.

The problem? Cost.

Using clinical dosages of effective ingredients gets really expensive, really fast. Instead of shaving their formulation down to a handful of properly dosed, effective ingredients, Shady Supplements goes in the opposite direction.

They decide to include miniscule amounts of substances proven to be effective in much larger dosages, and then throw in tiny amounts of a bunch of junk for good measure. Just like that, a new proprietary blend is born, and all they have to tell you is the total weight of everything in the blend, not of the individual ingredients themselves.

Another little trick of the proprietary blend is the fact that ingredients are listed in descending order according to predominance by weight, so when the first ingredient in a blend is something cheap, let's say malto-dextrin (a sweet, or sometimes tasteless, filler) or creatine monohydrate, it could be (and often is) 90%+ of the actual product.

No matter how many other ingredients are listed after the first, they could altogether only constitute a very small percentage of the actual blend.

Then Shady Supplement's marketing department gets ahold of the product and links it to all the benefits they can find, and often invent and embellish too, based on the ingredients that would be effective if the dosages weren't a mere fraction of the clinical dosages.

In the end, this means you pay $30 - 50 for something that cost Shady Supplements $5 to manufacture, and that would've cost $30 to create if the junk were dropped and clinical dosages were used for the worthwhile ingredients.

So the first thing you should demand as a consumer is no proprietary blends. There's absolutely no reason to use them for anything other than deception and fraud. All the science behind effective ingredients is publicly available. Everyone knows what works and doesn't, and in what dosages. Claims of "trade secrets" are bogus.

The second thing to know is that more ingredients doesn't mean a better product. In fact, you won't find a legitimate pre-workout with 30 ingredients because it's not financially feasible to include so many ingredients at clinically effective dosages (and you would be hard pressed to even find 30 ingredients worth using, period).

By choosing wisely, you can force the changes that need to happen: the death of the proprietary blend, the use of clinical dosages for effective ingredients, and the elimination of ineffective "label filler" ingredients.

So, this brings us back to the original question: pre-workout or caffeine pills?

Well, caffeine is a useful pre-workout stimulant that can increase muscle endurance and strength, but the fact is there are plenty of other safe, natural substances that can further improve your performance...if they're dosed properly.

So, all things considered, a good pre-workout supplement is worth the investment, in my opinion. It will give you a kick of energy, a good pump, and increased muscle endurance.

One thing you should know about pre-workout drinks, however, is that most contain quite a bit of caffeine per serving (anywhere from 100-300 mg). If your body is sensitive to caffeine, you might want to try one with little or no caffeine.

CREATINE

Creatine is a substance found naturally in the body and in foods like red meat. It is perhaps the most researched dietary supplement in the world of sports nutrition--the subject of over 200 studies.

Research has shown that supplementation with creatine can...

- Help build muscle and and improve strength[46-48]

- Improve anaerobic endurance[49, 50]

- Reduce muscle damage and soreness from exercise[51, 52]

And in case you're worried that creatine is bad for your kidneys, these claims have been categorically and repeatedly disproven[53, 54].

In healthy subjects, creatine has been shown to have no harmful side effects, in both short- or long-term usage[55-57]. People with kidney disease are not advised to supplement with creatine, however[58].

What type of creatine should you take though?

Creatine monohydrate has been the subject of the vast majority of studies done on the creatine molecule and is a proven winner, but the marketing machines of supplement companies are constantly pumping up fancy-sounding stuff like creatine citrate, creatine ethyl ester, liquid creatine, creatine nitrate, buffered creatine, creatine hydrochloride, and others.

These variations are certainly more *expensive* than creatine monohydrate, but are they any more *effective*? The short answer is NO, they're not.

Certain forms of creatine are more water soluble, such as creatine citrate[59], nitrate[60], and hydrochloride (the research backing this claim has disappeared, so I can't cite it), but this doesn't make them more effective in your body.

Don't overpay for over-hyped forms of creatine pushed by million-dollar ads and sold in fancy bottles. Creatine monohydrate is the best bang for your buck, and is the standard by which all other forms of creatine are still judged.

If creatine monohydrate bothers your stomach, try a more water soluble form of creatine such as micronized creatine, or creatine citrate, nitrate, or hydrocholoride.

HGH BOOSTERS

Most HGH (human growth hormone) boosters are a waste of money. They're usually full of amino acids that do provide various benefits when dosed properly, but which have never been proven to increase GH levels.

Another common ingredient is gamma aminobutyric acid, or GABA. Research has shown that supplementation with GABA elevates resting and postexercise growth hormone levels[61, 62], but the forms of GH increased have not been proven to contribute to muscle growth (there are over 100 forms of GH in your body, and all perform different functions).

Save your money and skip the HGH boosters.

GLUTAMINE

Glutamine is the most abundant amino acid in the body, and is heavily depleted by intense, prolonged exercise[63, 64].

Research has shown that supplementation with glutamine can...

- Reduce the negative effects of prolonged exercise on the immune system[65] (research has shown that exercise depletes glutamine levels in the body, which in turn can impair immune function[66, 67]).

- Improve your endurance and reduce fatigue in prolonged exercise[68, 69].

- Help your body better deal with the systemic stress of prolonged exercise[70-72].

While glutamine is a worthwhile supplement backed by good science, it's not without hype. And the claims usually revolve around building and preserving muscle. Can supplementation with glutamine do this?

Not quite.

Research has shown that intramuscular glutamine levels play an important role in protein synthesis[73] and the prevention of muscle breakdown[74], and glutamine does improve the body's ability to use leucine[75] (an essential amino acid that plays a vital role in protein synthesis).

That said, there are no studies to indicate that supplementation with glutamine improves protein synthesis in healthy, well-fed adults (as opposed to humans and rats in diseased or under-fed states).

To the contrary, in fact, several studies conducted with healthy adults showed that supplementation with glutamine has no effect on protein synthesis, muscle performance, body composition, or the prevention of muscle breakdown[76-78].

So, while supplementation with glutamine may not provide an anabolic boost, its anti-stress and anti-fatigue benefits make it a worthwhile buy if you're exercising regularly, intensely, and for prolonged periods.

NITRIC OXIDE SUPPLEMENTS

These supplements are commonly composed of the amino acids arginine, citrulline, and beta-alanine, with claims of stimulating the body's production of a substance called nitric oxide. Nitric oxide (NO) widens blood vessels and thus enables more oxygen and nutrients to get to the muscles (as the blood transports oxygen and nutrients).

While this sounds like another dubious marketing pitch, there are studies to support these claims[79-81], and I have found several of these products helpful.

That said, most pre-workout drinks these days contain these "NO-boosting" aminos though, so buying them separately isn't necessary. But if you're not taking a pre-workout, or your pre-workout drink doesn't contain arginine, citrulline, or beta-alanine, then you could benefit from a good (properly dosed) NO-booster.

MULTI-VITAMINS

Vitamins and minerals are necessary for many metabolic processes in the body and are important in supporting growth and development.

Vitamins and minerals also are required in numerous reactions involved with exercise and physical activity, including energy, carbohydrate, fat and protein metabolism, oxygen transfer and delivery, and tissue repair.

Deficiencies in key vitamins and minerals, such as B vitamins, vitamin C, iron, and magnesium, can cause many performance problems such as anemia, impaired muscle function and work capacity, and reduced aerobic and muscular endurance.

As you would expect, exercising increases your body's vitamin and mineral requirements, and as the intensity, duration, and frequency increases, so do your body's needs for micronutrients.

While research has shown that eating a variety of foods can provide adequate vitamins and minerals[82], achieving enough variety is often easier said than done when considering food preferences and availability.

For example:

- If you eat insufficient fruits and vegetables, you can become deficient in antioxidant nutrients such as vitamins A, E, and C, which play important roles in helping the body combat the oxidative stress of exercise.

- If you eat insufficient fish, beef, or poultry, an iron deficiency can develop. This leads to impaired muscle function and work capacity and, if uncorrected, this can lead to anemia, which can take 3 - 6 months to reverse.

- If you don't get enough zinc in your diet by eating foods such as beef, poultry, beans, dairy, and nuts, you can develop a zinc deficiency, which can impair its ability to build and repair muscle tissue and produce energy.

The story is the same for each of the essential vitamins and minerals: if your diet is low in a certain type of food, you're probably getting too little of one or more vitamins and minerals, which results in negative side effects. Further complicating the matter is the fact that several studies show a long-term, steady decline of micronutrients in our food due to soil depletion and agricultural practices designed to improve traits (size, growth rate, pest resistance) other than nutrition[83].

Unsurprisingly, then, research has shown that many athletes under-consume micronutrients, and thus can benefit from supplementation[84]. Further, your risk for vitamin and mineral deficiencies increases when you're restricting your calories (dieting to lose weight), making supplementation even more desirable under those conditions[85-87].

So, the bottom line is this:

If you eat substantial amount of a wide variety of foods every day, you may be getting everything you need in the way of vitamins and minerals from your food. But many people aren't, and supplementation can help provide what's missing.

I take a multi-vitamin every day for this reason, and recommend that you do too.

CLA

Conjugated linoleic acid, or CLA, is an essential fatty acid that occurs naturally in dairy products and meats.

Multiple studies have confirmed that supplementation with CLA helps reduce body fat and prevent weight gain[88-91], and also helps preserve muscle by lessening the catabolic effect of training on muscle protein[92].

Like any truly helpful fat loss supplement, CLA is no wonder product, but it does give a little boost to your fat loss regimen.

FAT BURNERS

The weight loss industry is HUGE (like $30 billion+ huge) and scams abound. It seems like a new "wonder ingredient" takes the media by storm every couple of months, and millions upon millions of dollars are quickly wasted on crap like acai berry drinks and resveratrol pills.

Many people incorrectly believe that a pill can trigger massive fat loss. This simply isn't true.

There are, however, certain "fat burner" supplements can help speed up the process of losing weight when you're dieting and training properly.

The most effective ones rely on caffeine and other stimulants to boost the metabolism, but you have a few other options too.there are a few other ingredients that can help too.

Instead of breaking down the various ingredients, just check out the fat burners I recommend in the bonus report. They're backed by sound science, and I've used them extensively and can confidently say that they work.

GREEN TEA EXTRACT

Green tea extract is an herbal product derived from green tea leaves. It contains a large amount of a substance known as a "catechin," which is responsible for many of tea's health benefits[93].

One of these benefits relates to weight loss. Research has shown that supplementation with GTE accelerates exercise-induced fat loss[94], and can help reduce abdominal fat[95], in particular.

GTE is an effective, inexpensive way to speed up your fat loss.

FISH OIL

Fish oil is a mixture of fatty acids, two of which provide substantial benefits to the body: eicosapentaenoic acid (EPA) and docosahexaenoic acid (DHA). These are known as "omega-3" fatty acids, and are considered "essential" fatty acids, meaning they can't be synthesized by the body— they must be obtained from the diet.

The two most popular types of omega-3 fatty acid supplements are fish oil and oil from the seeds of plants like flax, hemp, canola, and others, which contain alpha-linolenic acid. Fish oil is a superior source of omega-3s, due to the body's inefficient conversion of ALA into EPA and DHA[96, 97] (whereas fish oil directly contains EPA and DHA).

Research has shown that supplementation with fish oil can...

- Increase muscle protein synthesis[98, 99].

- Reduce muscle soreness[100], inflammation[101-103], and anxiety[104].

- Decrease blood pressure[105, 106], depression[107, 108], negative effects of stress[109, 110], and the risk for kidney and cardiovascular disease[111-113], as well as stroke[114] and metabolic syndrome[115].

- Improve glucose uptake and insulin sensitivity in people with impaired insulin metabolism, and preserve it in the metabolically healthy [116-118].

- Improve memory[119] and cognitive performance[120, 121].

- Prevent weight gain[122-124].

- Speed up fat loss[125-127].

Simply put, fish oil is an incredibly effective supplement for maintaining optimal health and performance, both in and out of the gym.

As with every other health and fitness supplement, not all fish oils are the same. There are two forms on the market today: the triglyceride form, and the ethyl ester form.

The triglyceride form is fish oil in its natural state, and the ethyl ester form is a processed version of the triglyceride form that includes a molecule of ethanol (alcohol)[128].

While plenty of studies have proven the benefits of supplementation with fatty acid ethyl esters (FAEEs), research has shown that the triglyceride form is better absorbed by the body[129-131]. One of the reasons for this is the ethyl ester form is much more resistant to the enzymatic process by which the body breaks the oil down for use[132].

Another downside to the ethyl ester form is during the digestive process, your body converts it back to the triglyceride form, which results in the release of the ethanol molecule. Although the dose is small, those with alcohol sensitivity or addiction can be negatively affected. Research has provided evidence of cellular and organic toxicity and injury resulting from the ingestion of FAEEs[133-137].

And in case you're worried that the triglyceride form contains more lead, mercury, PCBs, or other contaminants, research has proven this to be untrue[138-141].

So, I highly recommend regular supplementation with fish oil. Like a multivitamin, it's a great choice for preventing many health issues.

THE BOTTOM LINE

The above supplements are the most commonly advertised and sold. You will undoubtedly run across other types as you browse the shelves at your local supplement and vitamin store. Do your wallet a favor and skip 'em all—especially the super-fancy-sounding ones.

While you can make great gains without any supplements, if you're willing to spend some money to get the most out of your training, then I'd recommend the following supplements (and in this order, if you're going to get less than all):

- A protein powder
- A multi-vitamin
- Fish oil
- Creatine
- Glutamine

- A pre-workout drink
- Fat burner, CLA, and GTE (if dieting to lose weight)
- An NO booster

And again, check out the bonus report if you'd like to see which brands and products I specifically use and recommend.

22

THE *THINNER*
LEANER STRONGER
SUPPLEMENT ROUTINE

LET'S GO OVER HOW TO PROPERLY take each of the supplements I recommended in the previous chapter.

PROTEIN SUPPLEMENT

I like to use protein supplements before and after workouts, and in between my whole food meals. There's no set rule as to when or how often you should be taking protein supplements, but I find my body does best if I get at least 50% of my daily protein from whole food sources. Protein supplements are meant to be just that—supplements—and not primary sources of daily protein.

When using whey for post-workout nutrition, research has shown that 20 grams of protein is enough to stimulate maximal protein synthesis in young, healthy males[142]. As age increases, so does the amount of post-workout protein needed to stimulate maximal protein synthesis. In the elderly, for example, research showed that 35-40 grams stimulates more protein synthesis than 20 grams[143, 144].

Whey protein can also be used as an effective pre-workout supplement, as research has shown protein ingested 30 minutes prior to training can reduce muscle damage and soreness[145].

PRE-WORKOUT DRINKS

Take this about 30 minutes before your workout. The emptier your stomach is when you take it, the more you'll feel it.

CREATINE

The method most commonly used in clinical studies, and thus proven effective, is as follows:

1. For the first 5-7 days, you should take 20 grams of creatine daily, as this rapidly increases your body's total creatine content and storage[146, 147]. 4 separate servings of 5 grams each is the common method of achieving this.

2. After the "loading" phase, you should take a maintenance dose of 3-5 grams per day[146].

Research has shown that ingesting creatine with carbohydrates increases its accumulation in the muscles[148, 149], and thus it's recommended that you take it with meals containing carbohydrates.

Many experts also talk about the need to "cycle" your creatine (take it for a few months, stop for a month or two, begin again, and so forth). The reason given for this is the claim that when you're supplementing creatine, your body reduces its own production. By cycling it, you give your body a chance to reset its own creatine production. While this may be true, I've yet to find any studies that support it. I don't cycle creatine—I simply take 5 grams per day, every day.

Always take a serving with your post-workout meal, when it will get sucked right into the muscles due to the high amount of carbs in the meal. If you're doing 5 grams per day, do it after your workout. When loading, just make sure you get a serving after training.

GLUTAMINE

For you to derive benefits from glutamine supplementation, you must take enough each day, and research has shown that chronic usage is important[150].

Studies have shown dosages ranging between 5-30 grams per day to be both safe and beneficial[151], but 0.1-0.2 grams per kilogram of body weight per day has been shown to be sufficient for athletes[150, 152].

NITRIC OXIDE SUPPLEMENTS

If you want to try these out, just follow the instructions on the label.

MULTI-VITAMINS

Follow the instructions on the label. Most multis will have you take ½ of a serving with breakfast and ½ of a serving with dinner.

CLA

According to the CLA studies cited in the previous chapter, dosages of 3-7 grams per day are most effective. You should spread this out over three servings (one with breakfast, lunch, and dinner).

FAT BURNERS

Simply follow the directions, which vary depending on which you're taking.

Don't take more than one fat burner at a time—it'll put way too much stress on your system. Cut out all other caffeine from your diet when you're on fat burners, as you don't want to be overloading your body with caffeine every day.

GREEN TEA EXTRACT

Based on the studies cited earlier, you want to take 600-900 mg of catechins per day to realize their weight loss benefits. The average GTE product contains about 300 mg of catechins per pill.

FISH OIL

Research indicates that 3.5-4.5grams of fish oil per day is ideal for a person eating a normal, 2,000-calorie diet[153, 154], and that just over 6.5 grams per day is the upper limit recommended[154].

The range of 3-6 grams of fish oil per day is in line with the clinically effective dosages used in many of the studies proving the effectiveness of fish oil supplementation.

CONSISTENCY IS THE KEY

Just like training and diet, the most important aspect of supplementing is *consistency*. You must take your supplements consistently to realize the full benefits. You can't take creatine for a few days per week, forget on the other days, and expect much.

Fortunately, the supplements I recommend are easy to take in terms of schedule (a few times per day at the times when you're at home). But you need to make sure you follow the plan every day.

THE BOTTOM LINE

This chapter has just paid for the book probably a hundred times over (literally) because you're going to save hundreds of dollars each year (or more!) that you would've inevitably wasted on hyped-up junk products (trust me—you would've fallen into the trap like we all have).

Instead, you're going to spend your money efficiently and only on what is proven to give real, lasting gains. Just like the training philosophy of *Thinner Leaner Stronger* is "most results for your time and effort," the supplement philosophy is "most bang for your buck."

When you combine the simple supplement plan I just laid out with a complete, nutritious diet, you will enjoy maximum gains from your training.

23

FROM HERE, YOUR BODY WILL CHANGE

SO…I GUESS THIS IS it, right? We've reached the end…

No way.

You're in a process now—and yup, it's *already* begun—of proving to yourself that you *can* transform your body faster than you ever believed. Within your first 3-4 months of training, you're going to know with *absolute certainty* that you can follow what you've learned in this book to build the body of your dreams.

It's pretty cool to realize that you *do* have the power to change your body—to get thin, lean, strong, and healthy—and you are in control of your body, not the other way around.

No matter how "ordinary" you might think you are, I promise you that you can not only create an extraordinary body, but an extraordinary life as well. Don't be surprised if your newfound confidence and pride ripples out to affect other areas of your life too, inspiring you to reach for other goals and improve in other ways.

From here, all you have to do is walk the path I've laid out, and in twelve weeks, you'll look in the mirror and think, "I'm glad I did," not, "I wish I had."

My goal is to help you reach your goals, and I hope this book helps.

I want you to not only "get in shape" but to strive for achievements that you used to think impossible. I want you to feel confident, happy, and in control.

If we work together as a team, we can and will succeed.

So, I'd like you to make a promise as you begin your transformation: Can you promise me—and yourself—that you'll let me know when you've reached your goal?

You can find my contact information at the end of the book!

Oh and if you want to know where to go from here in terms of further educating yourself, I recommend you check out my book *Muscle Myths* next. In it, I address a whole new slew of myths and mistakes that keep people from getting the health and fitness results they want. It's the perfect companion to this book, and will build on the knowledge you now have.

For instance, in *Muscle Myths* you'll learn things like...

• The truth about the effects of fasting and the "starvation mode" myth. Yup, it's a myth, and you may even want to incorporate some fasting into your meal schedule.

• Why eating a substantial amount of carbohydrates every day won't make you fat as some "experts" claim, but why going low-carb can be beneficial for some.

• What you need to know about alcohol and its effects on your fat loss and muscle growth. (Hint: It's not nearly as bad as some people claim, and you don't have to totally abstain if you know what you're doing!)

• Why building muscle is one of the best things you can do to prevent the physical and mental decline associated with aging.

• The facts about how your sleep affects your fat loss, hormones, and muscle growth, and how to determine how much sleep your body really needs.

• Why the theory that stress and cortisol cause weight loss is bunk, and what you can do to help your body better deal with stress and stress hormones.

• And much more...

The bottom line is if you liked *Thinner Leaner Stronger*, you'll love *Muscle Myths*. As you would expect, every important claim and argument in the book is supported by both common sense and scientific literature (the book cites over 300 studies in all).

By the end, you'll have a whole new level of understanding of how the body works, and how to get the most out of your dieting and training.

Well, that's it for now. Thanks again for reading my book. I hope to hear from you soon, and good luck on your journey.

Q&A

Q: I CAN'T FIND TIME TO EXERCISE, BUT I WANT TO GET INTO SHAPE. WHAT CAN I DO?

A: I don't know anybody who can *find* time to exercise. I've never had anyone tell me, "Mike, I have too much free time these days. I think I'll just spend a few hours in the gym every day to get in shape. What should I do while I'm there?"

It's always the opposite: Most people lead busy, hectic lives, and they feel they don't have time for anything new. But that just isn't true. As much as most of us would like to *think* we're too busy to exercise, that's not the case.

People who have successfully transformed their bodies have only 24 hours in a day to do everything they need to do, just like you and me. And they have jobs, a family, a social life, and everything else to juggle. But here's the thing: They simply planned their days out and snuck in 45-60 minutes for exercise. Some watch an hour less of TV each night. Others wake up an hour early each day. Others get their spouses to handle their kids for an hour after dinner and use that time.

The point is that if you really want to work out the time, I'm positive you can do it.

Q: I TRAVEL A LOT. CAN I STILL FOLLOW THIS PROGRAM PROPERLY?

A: Absolutely, but it requires that you *plan*. Stay at hotels that are close to an adequate gym (pretty much all hotel exercise facilities are inadequate for the type of training you'll be doing) and plan when you'll work out. For most travelers, this means early in the morning or after dinner. Bring your supplements with you and just follow your regular routine.

Following a diet can be a bit tougher when traveling, but it can still be done. Before arriving, I find a nearby health food store (like Whole Foods) and plan out what to eat while visiting. When I arrive, I go stock up on what I need. If living a healthy, fulfilling life is a high enough priority for you, you can absolutely make it work.

If you're unable to make it to a gym while you're out of town, you can always do a bodyweight routine in your hotel room to help maintain your strength.

Here's what I do:

Push-ups to failure (one-handed if possible)

Rest 60 sec

Pull-ups to failure (I bring one of those bars that install in a doorway)

Rest 60 sec

Squats for 30 seconds (one-legged if possible)

Burpees for 30 seconds

Mountain climbers to failure

Rest 90 sec

Crunches to failure

Rest 60 sec

Start over with push-ups

I do this for 20-30 minutes, and find it very effective in keeping my strength and size up while I can't lift.

Q: I HURT MY (INSERT BODY PART HERE). WHAT SHOULD I DO?

Maintaining proper form and only working with weights you can correctly handle almost completely eliminates your chances of getting seriously injured. But, if you do happen to tweak something, there are a few things you should do to ensure it doesn't become more of a problem.

First is stay off whatever is hurting. If it's your shoulder, don't do any exercises that aggravate it, such as the Bench Press or Military Press. If it's your knee, lay off the Squats and Deadlifts. You want to give the affected part complete rest until it's fully better.

Alternating ice and heat can help markedly. What I've done is brought a microwavable heat pack and two ice packs to work, and just switched between them throughout the day (two ice packs so you can always have one ready).

Massage can work wonders with strained muscles, and chiropractic care can help with neck and back issues.

I've also found that stretching and foam rolling can help by loosening up the muscles affected (which are almost always tense), and by increasing blood flow to the area, thereby improving recovery.

Once the area seems to be fully healed up (no more pain, and you can move the muscles through their normal ranges of motion), I recommend that you ease back into the exercises that directly stress it. Work in the 12-15 rep range for your first week and ensure that everything feels fine before you load up the weights again.

Please note that the above recommendations are for strains and tweaks. If you're in excruciating pain and it just won't go away, then you should see a doctor.

Q: I SHOWED THIS BOOK TO A TRAINER, AND HE DIDN'T LIKE IT AND SAID I SHOULD DO SOMETHING ELSE. IS HE RIGHT?

A: I'm sure the trainer's heart is in the right place and he's just trying to help, but unfortunately most trainers just don't know what they're talking about. Most aren't even in great shape themselves and are just teaching whatever they learned in their textbooks without knowing if the methods they are teaching are actually the most effective or not.

If you follow what I wrote in this book, you *will* make awesome gains—I guarantee you that. Tens, if not hundreds, of thousands of people around the world follow routines just like this, and their results speak for themselves.

Q: HOW MUCH WEIGHT CAN I GAIN OR LOSE WITH THIS PROGRAM AND HOW QUICKLY?

A: I've been helping people with this system for many years, and most women can gain around 5 pounds of muscle or lose between 10-15 pounds of fat in their first 3 months. If you're gaining more than 2 pounds per week, you're gaining more fat than is necessary. If you're losing more than 2 pounds per week, you may be losing too much muscle, which can be a problem in the long run.

Q: I HAVE A LOT OF TROUBLE GAINING MUSCLE. WILL THIS PROGRAM WORK FOR ME?

A: Absolutely. I don't believe in the "hardgainer" myth. In my many years in this game, I've never met a "hardgainer" that was actually training and eating properly. In most cases, they weren't lifting for maximum muscle gains and weren't eating enough.

I promise you that if you train how I say to train and eat how I say to eat, you will gain muscle. End of story.

Q: I'M SICK. SHOULD I TRY TO TRAIN ANYWAY?

A: As much as you might want to, don't. I've made this mistake many times and it only drags the sickness out. Just take it easy, get well, and get back on track.

Q: I HAVE TROUBLE WITH PREPARING HEALTHY MEALS THROUGHOUT THE WEEK. WHAT SHOULD I DO?

A: A simple solution is to prepare healthy meals in batches and then portion them out, and bring them to work with you. Pop it in a toaster oven or microwave for a few minutes, and you're good to go.

When I do this, I prepare a few day's worth of food at a time, so I'll cook a batch up on Sundays and Wednesdays.

Q: MY OUT-OF-SHAPE FRIENDS ALWAYS WANT ME TO EAT UNHEALTHY STUFF WITH THEM. WHAT SHOULD I DO?

A: Don't fall into the trap that made them out of shape in the first place. When you eat with people who don't eat well, you should be careful to not use their poor habits as justification for you to follow suit.

You can also try to inspire them to join you in your quest for a healthier, more energetic, and better-looking body. Or, if necessary, only eat with them when you can have a cheat meal.

Q: I'VE BEEN UNABLE TO STICK WITH WORKOUT PROGRAMS. WHY SHOULD I EVEN TRY YOURS?

A: Nothing is more annoying than working your butt off in the gym every day and seeing no results. This is, hands down, the number one reason why people quit their workout routines. Well, this program works. And, better yet, it works quickly.

Imagine if, in 3 months, you've lost 20 pounds of fat and built lean, toned muscle that shows. Imagine if your friends and family keep commenting on how good you look. Guys start turning their heads. Women you know are asking what in the world you're doing. You feel strong and energetic—better than you have in a long time.

Well, that's totally achievable. All you have to do is get started.

Q: I'M GOING TO BE OUT OF TOWN AND WON'T HAVE ACCESS TO A GYM. HOW SHOULD I EAT?

A: If your trip is going to be a week or less, just eat normally, as the effects of a week of no training are negligible.

If your trip is going to be longer than a week, however, then I recommend that you do a bodyweight routine, and try not to go overboard on the eating (I could tell you to work out your maintenance diet and follow that while you're gone, but that probably wouldn't be practical).

A simple routine you can do when on the road to maintain muscle mass is a circuit of pull-ups, push-up, squats, and burpees. Mine is very simple: I do as many pull-ups as I can, rest thirty seconds, and then do as many push-ups as I can, rest thirty seconds, and then do as many squats as I can, rest thirty seconds, and do as many burpees as I can. I then rest 2-3 minutes and do it all again. I do this circuit 4-6 times and I'm toast.

(To do this, I bring a disassembled pull-up bar and assemble it in my hotel room. You can find the one I use on my website, www.muscleforlife.com, under in the Recommendations section.)

BONUS REPORT

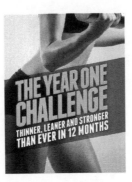

EXACTLY HOW TO TRAIN AND EAT TO GET INTO THE BEST SHAPE OF YOUR LIFE...IN YOUR FIRST YEAR! PEOPLE WON'T BELIEVE THEIR EYES!

Would you like a full, detailed training program to follow for the next year to ensure that you get thinner, leaner, and stronger than ever?

You now know things that most women will never understand about how to build a lean, strong, and healthy body, but you might feel a bit unsure about how to create your workouts, which brands of supplements to buy, what gear is best, and so on.

Well, thanks to feedback from hundreds of readers, I created this totally free bonus report to help you out. In it, I cover things like...

- What brands of supplements I recommend and why. I've tried pretty much every brand you can name over the years, and have found what I feel are the best of the best for each type of supplement that I recommend.

- The workout equipment that is actually useful, and the brands that have stood the test of time for me. I've torn through gloves, tried all kinds of crappy straps, tried every body fat testing device you can buy, and even tried many types of shakers, and I want to save you the money and frustration of buying junk.

- Complete workout plans for your entire first year of training. All you'll have to do is show up every day and do what I say, and you'll get thinner, leaner, and stronger faster than ever.

- 8 delicious recipes from my cookbook, *The Shredded Chef: 120 Recipes for Building Muscle, Getting Lean, and Staying Healthy.*

- And more!

By following this program, you're going to build a physique that you're proud of. It will be a trophy for your unswerving dedication, perseverance, and toughness.

My mission is to help you get to that moment. That's what makes me most happy.

Download this free special report today and make this next year the year where you get thinner, leaner, and stronger than ever!

Visit WWW.BIT.LY/TLS-YEAR-ONE to get this report now!

WOULD YOU DO ME A FAVOR?

Thank you for buying my book. I'm positive that if you just follow what I've written, you will be on your way to looking and feeling better than you ever have before.

I have a small favor to ask. Would you mind taking a minute to write a blurb on Amazon about this book? I check all my reviews and love to get feedback (that's the real pay for my work—knowing that I'm helping people).

Visit the following URL to leave me a review:

WWW.AMZN.TO/TLSREVIEW

Also, if you have any friends or family who might enjoy this book, spread the love and lend it to them!

Now, I don't just want to sell you a book—I want to see you use what you've learned to build the body of your dreams.

As you work toward your goals, however, you'll probably have questions or run into some difficulties. I'd like to be able to help you with these, so let's connect up! I don't charge for the help, of course, and I answer questions from readers every day.

Here's how we can connect:

Facebook: facebook.com/muscleforlifefitness

Twitter: @muscleforlife

G+: gplus.to/MuscleForLife

And last but not least, my website is www.muscleforlife.com and if you want to write me, my email address is mike@muscleforlife.com.

Thanks again and I wish you the best!

Mike

P.S. Turn to the next page to check out other books of mine that you might like!

NO PROPRIETARY BLENDS... NO PSEUDOSCIENCE... NO UNDERDOSING KEY INGREDIENTS... REAL WORKOUT SUPPLEMENTS THAT WORK!

HERE'S THE BOTTOM-LINE TRUTH OF THIS MULTI-BILLION-DOLLAR INDUSTRY:

While certain supplements can help, they do NOT build great physiques (proper training and nutrition does), and most are a complete waste of money.

Too many products are "proprietary blends" of low-quality ingredients, junk fillers, and unnecessary additives. Key ingredients are horribly underdosed. There's a distinct lack of credible scientific evidence to back up the outrageous claims made on labels and in ads. The list of what's wrong with this industry goes on and on.

And that's why I decided to get into the supplement game.

What gives? Am I just a hypocritical sell-out? Well, hear me out for a minute and then decide. The last thing we need is yet another marketing machine churning out yet another line of hyped up, flashy products claiming to be more effective than steroids.

I think things should be done differently, and that's why I started LEGION.

Here's what sets LEGION apart from the rabble:

✔ **100% transparent product formulas**

The only reason to use proprietary blends is fraud and deception. You deserve to know exactly what you're buying.

✔ **100% science-based ingredients and dosages**

Every ingredient we use is backed by published scientific literature and is included at true clinically effective dosages.

✔ **100% naturally sweetened with stevia**

Research suggests that regular consumption of artificial sweeteners can be harmful to our health, which is why we use stevia, a natural sweetener with proven health benefits.

LEGION SUPPLEMENTS ARE NOT ONLY A BETTER VALUE AND BETTER FOR YOUR HEALTH… THEY DELIVER REAL RESULTS YOU CAN ACTUALLY FEEL.

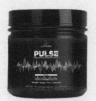

PULSE

PULSE provides you with clinically effective dosages of caffeine, theanine, citrulline malate, beta-alanine, ornithine, and betaine. It's so good that you'll never want to use another pre-workout again.

WHEY+

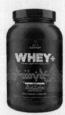

WHEY+ is 100% whey protein isolate (which means no upset stomachs), naturally sweetened, and hormone-free, and has added leucine to further stimulate protein synthesis.

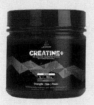

CREATINE+

CREATINE+ provides you with clinically effective dosages of micronized creatine monohydrate and fenugreek extract, which helps you build more muscle and strength and helps optimize your hormones.

RECHARGE

RECHARGE provides you with clinically effective dosages of L-glutamine and L-carnitine L-tartrate, which have been proven to improve muscle recovery, reduce fatigue, and fight off overtraining.

ORDER NOW AT
WWW.LEGIONSUPPLEMENTS.COM
AND SAVE 10%

ALSO BY MICHAEL MATTHEWS

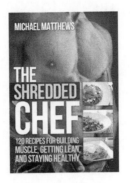

The Shredded Chef: 120 Recipes for Building Muscle, Getting Lean, and Staying Healthy

If you want to know how to forever escape the dreadful experience of "dieting" and learn how to cook nutritious, delicious meals that make building muscle and burning fat easy and enjoyable, then you need to read this book.

Visit www.muscleforlife.com to learn more about this book!

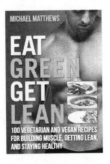

Eat Green Get Lean: 100 Vegetarian and Vegan Recipes for Building Muscle, Getting Lean, and Staying Healthy

If you want to know how to build muscle and burn fat by eating delicious vegetarian and vegan meals that are easy to cook and easy on your wallet, then you want to read this book.

Visit www.muscleforlife.com to learn more about this book!

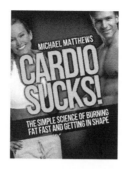

Cardio Sucks! The Simple Science of Burning Fat Fast and Getting in Shape

If you're short on time and sick of the same old boring cardio routine and want to kick your fat loss into high gear by working out less and...heaven forbid...actually have some fun...then you want to read this new book.

Visit www.muscleforlife.com to learn more about this book!

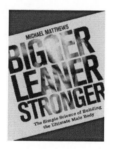

Bigger Leaner Stronger: The Simple Science of Building the Ultimate Male Body

If you want to be muscular, lean, and strong as quickly as possible, without steroids, good genetics, or wasting ridiculous amounts of time in the gym, and money on supplements...then you want to read this book.

Visit www.muscleforlife.com to learn more about this book!

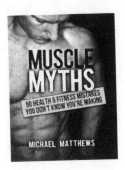

Muscle Myths: 50 Health & Fitness Mistakes You Don't Know You're Making

If you've ever felt lost in the sea of contradictory training and diet advice out there and you just want to know once and for all what works and what doesn't—what's scientifically true and what's false—when it comes to building muscle and getting ripped, then you need to read this book.

Visit www.muscleforlife.com to learn more about this book!

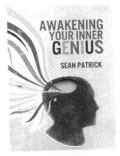

Awakening Your Inner Genius

If you'd like to know what some of history's greatest thinkers and achievers can teach you about awakening your inner genius, and how to find, follow, and fulfill your journey to greatness, then you want to read this book today.

(I'm using a pen name for this book, as well as for a few other projects not related to health and fitness, but I thought you might enjoy it so I'm including it here.)

Visit www.yourinnergenius.com to learn more about this book!

REFERENCES

1. Daniel W. D. West and Stuart M. Phillips.Associations of exercise-induced hormone profiles and gains in strength and hypertrophy in a large cohort after weight training.Eur J Appl Physiol. 2012 July; 112(7): 2693–2702.

2. Uchida MC, Crewther BT, Ugrinowitsch C, Bacurau RF, Moriscot AS, Aoki MS. Hormonal responses to different resistance exercise schemes of similar total volume. J Strength Cond Res. 2009 Oct;23(7):2003-8. doi: 10.1519/JSC.0b013e3181b73bf7.

3. Rogers et al. The Effect of Supplemental Isolated Weight-Training Exercises on Upper-Arm Size and Upper-Body Strength Human Performance Laboratory, Ball State University, Muncie, IN. NSCA Conference Abstract (2000).

4. Rhea MR, Alvar BA, Burkett LN, Ball SD. A meta-analysis to determine the dose response for strength development.Med Sci Sports Exerc. 2003 Mar;35(3):456-64.

5. Campos, Gerson E., et al. "Muscular adaptations in response to three different resistance-training regimens: specificity of repetition maximum training zones." European journal of applied physiology 88.1-2 (2002): 50-60.

6. E Jequier, K Acheson, and Y Schutz. Assessment of Energy Expenditure and Fuel Utilization in Man Annual Review of NutritionVol. 7: 187-208 (Volume publication date July 1987)DOI: 10.1146/annurev.nu.07.070187.001155.

7. Bellisle, France, Regina McDevitt, and Andrew M. Prentice. "Meal frequency and energy balance." British Journal of Nutrition 77.S1 (1997): S57-S70.

8. Cameron, Jameason D., Marie-Josée Cyr, and Éric Doucet. "Increased meal frequency does not promote greater weight loss in subjects who were prescribed an 8-week equi-energetic energy-restricted diet." British Journal of Nutrition 103.8 (2010): 1098.

9. Anderson, Jennifer Shultz. SEX DIFFERENCES IN THE RELATIONSHIP OF POLYUNSATURATED FATTY ACIDS AND NONINVASIVE IMAGING MEASURES OF SUBCLINICAL CARDIOVASCULAR DISEASE. Diss. Wake Forest University, 2011.

10. Young VR, Pellett PL. Plant proteins in relation to human protein and amino acid nutrition. Am J ClinNutr. 1994 May;59(5 Suppl):1203S-1212S.

11. Hwang, Chang Sun, et al. "Isoflavone metabolites and their< i> in vitro</i> dual functions: They can act as an estrogenic agonist or antagonist depending on the estrogen concentration." The Journal of steroid biochemistry and molecular biology 101.4 (2006): 246-253.

12. Kalman, Douglas, et al. "Effect of protein source and resistance training on body composition and sex hormones." Journal of the International Society of Sports Nutrition 4.1 (2007): 1-8.

13. Pennings B, Boirie Y, Senden JM, Gijsen AP, Kuipers H, van Loon LJ. Whey protein stimulates postprandial muscle protein accretion more effectively than do casein and casein hydrolysate in older men. Am J ClinNutr. 2011 May;93(5):997-1005. doi: 10.3945/ajcn.110.008102. Epub 2011 Mar 2.

14. Res, Peter T., et al. "Protein Ingestion before Sleep Improves Postexercise Overnight Recovery." Medicine and science in sports and exercise 44.8 (2012): 1560-1569.

15. Roberto Lanzi, LivioLuzi, Andrea Caumo, Anna Claudia Andreotti, Marco Federico Manzoni, Maria Elena Malighetti, Lucia PiceniSereni, Antonio EttorePontiroli. Elevated insulin levels contribute to the reduced growth hormone (GH) response to GH-releasing hormone in obese subjects. Metabolism Volume 48, Issue 9, September 1999, Pages 1152–1156.

16. J P Cappon, E Ipp, J A Brasel and D M Cooper. Acute effects of high fat and high glucose meals on the growth hormone response to exercise. doi: 10.1210/jc.76.6.1418 The Journal of Clinical Endocrinology & Metabolism June 1, 1993 vol. 76 no. 6 1418-1422 Department of Pediatrics, Harbor-UCLA Medical Center, Torrance 90509.

17. Chris Poole, Colin Wilborn, Lem Taylor and Chad Kerksick.THE ROLE OF POST-EXERCISE NUTRIENT ADMINISTRATION ON MUSCLE PROTEIN SYNTHESIS AND GLYCOGEN SYNTHESIS.© Journal of Sports Science and Medicine (2010) 9, 354 – 363.

18. Beelen, Milou, et al. "Nutritional strategies to promote postexercise recovery." International journal of sport nutrition and exercise metabolism 20.6 (2010): 515-532.

19. Res, Peter T., et al. "Protein ingestion prior to sleep improves post-exercise overnight recovery." Medicine and science in sports and exercise 44.4 (2012): 692-700.

20. Opland, Darren M., Gina M. Leinninger, and Martin G. Myers Jr. "Modulation of the mesolimbic dopamine system by leptin." Brain research 1350 (2010): 65-70.

21. Katzeff, Harvey L., et al. "Metabolic studies in human obesity during overnutrition and undernutrition: thermogenic and hormonal responses to norepinephrine." Metabolism 35.2 (1986): 166-175.

22. Jéquier, Eric. "Leptin signaling, adiposity, and energy balance." Annals of the New York Academy of Sciences 967.1 (2002): 379-388.

23. Dirlewanger, M., et al. "Effects of short-term carbohydrate or fat overfeeding on energy expenditure and plasma leptin concentrations in healthy female subjects." International journal of obesity 24.11 (2000): 1413-1418.

24. Bray, George A., et al. "Effect of dietary protein content on weight gain, energy expenditure, and body composition during overeating." JAMA: the journal of the American Medical Association 307.1 (2012): 47-55.

25. Röjdmark, S., J. Calissendorff, and K. Brismar. "Alcohol ingestion decreases both diurnal and nocturnal secretion of leptin in healthy individuals." Clinical endocrinology 55.5 (2001): 639-647.

26. Hawley JA. Molecular responses to strength and endurance training: are they incompatible? ApplPhysiolNutrMetab. 2009 Jun;34(3):355-61. doi: 10.1139/H09-023.

27. Nader GA. Concurrent strength and endurance training: from molecules to man. Med Sci Sports Exerc. 2006 Nov;38(11):1965-70.

28. Leveritt M, Abernethy PJ, Barry BK, Logan PA. Concurrent strength and endurance training.A review. Sports Med. 1999 Dec;28(6):413-27.

29. Häkkinen K, Alen M, Kraemer WJ, Gorostiaga E, Izquierdo M, Rusko H, Mikkola J, Häkkinen A, Valkeinen H, Kaarakainen E, Romu S, Erola V, Ahtiainen J, PaavolainenL.Neuromuscular adaptations during concurrent strength and endurance training versus strength training. Eur J Appl Physiol. 2003 Mar;89(1):42-52. Epub 2002 Dec 14.

30. Tremblay A, Simoneau JA, Bouchard C.Impact of exercise intensity on body fatness and skeletal muscle metabolism.Metabolism. 1994 Jul;43(7):814-8.

31. King, J. W. A comparison of the effects of interval training vs. continuous training on weight loss and body composition in obese pre-menopausal women (thesis).East Tennessee State University, 2001.

32. Treuth MS, Hunter GR, Williams M: Effects of exercise intensity on 24-h energy expenditure and substrate oxidation. Med Sci Sports Exerc28 :1138– 1143,1996.

33. Trapp EG, Chisholm DJ, Freund J, Boutcher SH. The effects of high-intensity intermittent exercise training on fat loss and fasting insulin levels of young women.Int J Obes (Lond). 2008 Apr;32(4):684-91. doi: 10.1038/sj.ijo.0803781. Epub 2008 Jan 15.

34. La Torre, Antonio, et al. "Acute effects of static stretching on squat jump performance at different knee starting angles." The Journal of Strength & Conditioning Research 24.3 (2010): 687-694.

35. Thacker, Stephen B., et al. "The impact of stretching on sports injury risk: a systematic review of the literature." Medicine & Science in Sports & Exercise 36.3 (2004): 371-378.

36. Rieu, Isabelle, et al. "Increased availability of leucine with leucine-rich whey proteins improves postprandial muscle protein synthesis in aging rats." Nutrition 23.4 (2007): 323-331.

37. Fujita, Satoshi, et al. "Nutrient signalling in the regulation of human muscle protein synthesis." The Journal of physiology 582.2 (2007): 813-823.

38. Frid AH, Nilsson M, Holst JJ, Björck IM.Effect of whey on blood glucose and insulin responses to composite breakfast and lunch meals in type 2 diabetic subjects.Am J ClinNutr. 2005 Jul;82(1):69-75.

39. Dangin, Martial, et al. "The digestion rate of protein is an independent regulating factor of postprandial protein retention." American Journal of Physiology-Endocrinology And Metabolism 280.2 (2001): E340-E348.

40. Pennings, Bart, et al. "Whey protein stimulates postprandial muscle protein accretion more effectively than do casein and casein hydrolysate in older men." The American journal of clinical nutrition 93.5 (2011): 997-1005.

41. Farrell Jr, H. M., et al. "Nomenclature of the proteins of cows' milk—sixth revision." Journal of Dairy Science 87.6 (2004): 1641-1674.

42. Potier, Mylne, and Daniel Tom. "Comparison of digestibility and quality of intact proteins with their respective hydrolysates." Journal of AOAC International 91.4

(2008): 1002-1005.

43. http://www.fda.gov/downloads/NewsEvents/MeetingsConferencesWorkshops/UCM1 63645.ppt.

44. Williams, Melvin H. "Facts and fallacies of purported ergogenic amino acid supplements." Clinics in sports medicine 18.3 (1999): 633-649.

45. http://www.fda.gov/food/guidancecomplianceregulatoryinformation/guidance documents/dietarysupplements/dietarysupplementlabelingguide/ucm070597. htm#4-34

46. Branch, J. David. "Effect of creatine supplementation on body composition and performance: a meta-analysis." International journal of sport nutrition and exercise metabolism 13.2 (2003): 198.

47. Law, Yu Li Lydia, et al. "Effects of two and five days of creatine loading on muscular strength and anaerobic power in trained athletes." The Journal of Strength & Conditioning Research 23.3 (2009): 906-914.

48. Rawson, ERIC S., and JEFF S. Volek. "Effects of creatine supplementation and resistance training on muscle strength and weightlifting performance." Journal of Strength and Conditioning Research 17.4 (2003): 822-831.

49. Eckerson, JOAN M., et al. "Effect of creatine phosphate supplementation on anaerobic working capacity and body weight after two and six days of loading in men and women." Journal of Strength and Conditioning Research 19.4 (2005): 756.

50. Kocak, S., and Ü. Karli. "Effects of high dose oral creatine supplementation on anaerobic capacity of elite wrestlers." Journal of sports medicine and physical fitness 43.4 (2003): 488-492.

51. Bassit, Reinaldo Abunasser, et al. "Effect of short-term creatine supplementation on markers of skeletal muscle damage after strenuous contractile activity." European journal of applied physiology 108.5 (2010): 945-955.

52. Santos, R. V. T., et al. "The effect of creatine supplementation upon inflammatory and muscle soreness markers after a 30km race." Life sciences 75.16 (2004): 1917-1924.

53. Poortmans JR, Francaux M. Adverse effects of creatine supplementation: fact or fiction? Sports Med. 2000 Sep;30(3):155-70.

54. Terjung RL, Clarkson P, Eichner ER, Greenhaff PL, Hespel PJ, Israel RG, Kraemer WJ, Meyer RA, Spriet LL, Tarnopolsky MA, Wagenmakers AJ, Williams MH. American College of Sports Medicine roundtable. The physiological and health effects of oral creatine supplementation. Med Sci Sports Exerc. 2000 Mar;32(3):706-17.

55. Yoshizumi WM, Tsourounis C. Effects of creatine supplementation on renal function. J Herb Pharmacother. 2004;4(1):1-7.

56. Bizzarini E, De Angelis L. Is the use of oral creatine supplementation safe? J Sports Med Phys Fitness. 2004 Dec;44(4):411-6.

57. Groeneveld GJ, Beijer C, Veldink JH, Kalmijn S, Wokke JH, van den Berg LH. Few adverse effects of long-term creatine supplementation in a placebo-controlled trial. Int J Sports Med. 2005 May;26(4):307-13.

58. Francaux M, Poortmans JR. Side effects of creatine supplementation in athletes. Int J

Sports Physiol Perform. 2006 Dec;1(4):311-23.

59. Jäger R, Harris RC, Purpura M, Francaux M. Comparison of new forms of creatine in raising plasma creatine levels. J IntSoc Sports Nutr. 2007 Nov 12;4:17.

60. A. Pandit, P. Mistry, P. Dib, A. Nikolaidis, A. K. Dash. EQUILIBRIUM SOLUBILTY STUDIES OF CREATINE NITRATE, CREATINE MONOHYDRATE AND BUFFERED CREATINE.

61. Powers ME, Yarrow JF, McCoy SC, Borst SE. Growth hormone isoform responses to GABA ingestion at rest and after exercise. Med Sci Sports Exerc. 2008 Jan;40(1):104-10.

62. Cavagnini F, Invitti C, Pinto M, Maraschini C, Di Landro A, Dubini A, Marelli A. Effect of acute and repeated administration of gamma aminobutyric acid (GABA) on growth hormone and prolactin secretion in man. ActaEndocrinol (Copenh). 1980 Feb;93(2):149-54.

63. Robson, PJet, et al. "Effects of exercise intensity, duration and recovery on in vitro neutrophil function in male athletes." International journal of sports medicine 20 (1999): 128-135.

64. Babij, P., S. M. Matthews, and M. J. Rennie. "Changes in blood ammonia, lactate and amino acids in relation to workload during bicycle ergometer exercise in man." European journal of applied physiology and occupational physiology 50.3 (1983): 405-411.

65. Castell, Linda M. "Can glutamine modify the apparent immunodepression observed after prolonged, exhaustive exercise?." Nutrition 18.5 (2002): 371-375.

66. Parry-Billings, M. A. R. K., et al. "Plasma amino acid concentrations in the overtraining syndrome: possible effects on the immune system." Medicine and science in sports and exercise 24.12 (1992): 1353.

67. Calder, P. C., and P. Yaqoob. "Glutamine and the immune system." Amino acids 17.3 (1999): 227-241.

68. Carvalho-Peixoto, Jacqueline Carvalho-Peixoto J., Robson Cardilo Alves RC Alves, and L-C. Cameron Luiz-Claudio Cameron. "Glutamine and carbohydrate supplements reduce ammonemia increase during endurance field exercise." Applied Physiology, Nutrition, and Metabolism 32.6 (2007): 1186-1190.

69. Favano, Alessandra, et al. "Peptide glutamine supplementation for tolerance of intermittent exercise in soccer players." CLINICS-UNIVERSIDADE DE SAO PAULO- 63.1 (2008): 27.

70. Kingsbury, K. J., L. Kay, and M. Hjelm. "Contrasting plasma free amino acid patterns in elite athletes: association with fatigue and infection." British journal of sports medicine 32.1 (1998): 25-32.

71. Cruzat, Vinicius Fernandes, Marcelo Macedo Rogero, and Julio Tirapegui. "Effects of supplementation with free glutamine and the dipeptide alanyl-glutamine on parameters of muscle damage and inflammation in rats submitted to prolonged exercise." Cell biochemistry and function 28.1 (2010): 24-30.

72. Bassini-Cameron, Adriana, et al. "Glutamine protects against increases in blood ammonia in football players in an exercise intensity-dependent way." British

journal of sports medicine 42.4 (2008): 260-266.

73. Jepson, M. M., et al. "Relationship between glutamine concentration and protein synthesis in rat skeletal muscle." American Journal of Physiology-Endocrinology And Metabolism 255.2 (1988): E166-E172.

74. MacLennan, Peter A., et al. "Inhibition of protein breakdown by glutamine in perfused rat skeletal muscle." FEBS letters 237.1 (1988): 133-136.

75. Hankard, REGIS G., MOREY W. Haymond, and D. O. M. I. N. I. Q. U. E. Darmaun. "Effect of glutamine on leucine metabolism in humans." American Journal of Physiology-Endocrinology And Metabolism 271.4 (1996): E748-E754.

76. Antonio, J. O. S. E., et al. "The effects of high-dose glutamine ingestion on weightlifting performance." Journal of strength and conditioning research 16.1 (2002): 157-160.

77. Candow, Darren G., et al. "Effect of glutamine supplementation combined with resistance training in young adults." European journal of applied physiology 86.2 (2001): 142-149.

78. Wilkinson, Sarah B. Wilkinson SB, et al. "Addition of glutamine to essential amino acids and carbohydrate does not enhance anabolism in young human males following exercise." Applied Physiology, Nutrition, and Metabolism 31.5 (2006): 518-529.

79. Álvares TS, Meirelles CM, Bhambhani YN, Paschoalin VM, Gomes PS. L-Arginine as a potential ergogenic aid in healthy subjects. Sports Med. 2011 Mar 1;41(3):233-48. doi: 10.2165/11538590-000000000-00000.

80. Sureda A, Cordova A, Ferrer MD, Tauler P, Perez G, Tur JA, Pons A. Effects of L-citrulline oral supplementation on polymorphonuclear neutrophils oxidative burst and nitric oxide production after exercise. Free Radic Res. 2009 Sep;43(9):828-35. doi: 10.1080/10715760903071664. Epub 2009 Jul 6.

81. Artioli GG, Gualano B, Smith A, Stout J, Lancha AH Jr. Role of beta-alanine supplementation on muscle carnosine and exercise performance. Med Sci Sports Exerc. 2010 Jun;42(6):1162-73. doi: 10.1249/MSS.0b013e3181c74e38.

82. American Dietetic Association; Dietitians of Canada; American College of Sports Medicine, Rodriguez NR, Di Marco NM, Langley S. American College of Sports Medicine position stand. Nutrition and athletic performance. Med Sci Sports Exerc. 2009 Mar;41(3):709-31. doi: 10.1249/MSS.0b013e31890eb86.

83. http://www.scientificamerican.com/article.cfm?id=soil-depletion-and-nutrition-loss.

84. Volpe SL. Micronutrient requirements for athletes. Clin Sports Med. 2007 Jan;26(1):119-30.

85. American Dietetic Association; Dietitians of Canada; American College of Sports Medicine, Rodriguez NR, Di Marco NM, Langley S. American College of Sports Medicine position stand. Nutrition and athletic performance. Med Sci Sports Exerc. 2009 Mar;41(3):709-31. doi: 10.1249/MSS.0b013e31890eb86.

86. Lukaski HC. Vitamin and mineral status: effects on physical performance. Nutrition. 2004 Jul-Aug;20(7-8):632-44.

87. Volpe SL. Micronutrient requirements for athletes. Clin Sports Med. 2007 Jan;26(1):119-30.

88. Gaullier JM, Halse J, Høye K, Kristiansen K, Fagertun H, Vik H, Gudmundsen O. Conjugated linoleic acid supplementation for 1 y reduces body fat mass in healthy overweight humans. Am J ClinNutr. 2004 Jun;79(6):1118-25.

89. Gaullier JM, Halse J, Høye K, Kristiansen K, Fagertun H, Vik H, Gudmundsen O. Supplementation with conjugated linoleic acid for 24 months is well tolerated by and reduces body fat mass in healthy, overweight humans. J Nutr. 2005 Apr;135(4):778-84.

90. Watras AC, Buchholz AC, Close RN, Zhang Z, Schoeller DA. The role of conjugated linoleic acid in reducing body fat and preventing holiday weight gain. Int J Obes (Lond). 2007 Mar;31(3):481-7. Epub 2006 Aug 22.

91. Whigham LD, Watras AC, Schoeller DA. Efficacy of conjugated linoleic acid for reducing fat mass: a meta-analysis in humans. Am J ClinNutr. 2007 May;85(5):1203-11.

92. Pinkoski C, Chilibeck PD, Candow DG, Esliger D, Ewaschuk JB, Facci M, Farthing JP, Zello GA. The effects of conjugated linoleic acid supplementation during resistance training. Med Sci Sports Exerc. 2006 Feb;38(2):339-48.

93. Yang, Chung S., Joshua D. Lambert, and Shengmin Sang. "Antioxidative and anticarcinogenic activities of tea polyphenols." Archives of toxicology 83.1 (2009): 11-21.

94. Venables, Michelle C., et al. "Green tea extract ingestion, fat oxidation, and glucose tolerance in healthy humans." The American journal of clinical nutrition 87.3 (2008): 778-784.

95. Maki, Kevin C., et al. "Green tea catechin consumption enhances exercise-induced abdominal fat loss in overweight and obese adults." The Journal of nutrition 139.2 (2009): 264-270.

96. Gerster H. Can adults adequately convert alpha-linolenic acid (18:3n-3) to eicosapentaenoic acid (20:5n-3) and docosahexaenoic acid (22:6n-3)? Int J Vitam Nutr Res. 1998;68(3):159-73.

97. Brenna JT. Efficiency of conversion of alpha-linolenic acid to long chain n-3 fatty acids in man. Curr Opin Clin Nutr Metab Care. 2002 Mar;5(2):127-32.

98. Smith GI, Atherton P, Reeds DN, Mohammed BS, Rankin D, Rennie MJ, Mittendorfer B. Dietary omega-3 fatty acid supplementation increases the rate of muscle protein synthesis in older adults: a randomized controlled trial. Am J Clin Nutr. 2011 Feb;93(2):402-12. doi: 10.3945/ajcn.110.005611. Epub 2010 Dec 15.

99. Smith GI, Atherton P, Reeds DN, Mohammed BS, Rankin D, Rennie MJ, Mittendorfer B. Omega-3 polyunsaturated fatty acids augment the muscle protein anabolic response to hyperinsulinaemia-hyperaminoacidaemia in healthy young and middle-aged men and women. Clin Sci (Lond). 2011 Sep;121(6):267-78. doi: 10.1042/CS20100597.

100. Tartibian B, Maleki BH, Abbasi A. The effects of ingestion of omega-3 fatty acids on perceived pain and external symptoms of delayed onset muscle soreness in untrained men. Clin J Sport Med. 2009 Mar;19(2):115-9. doi: 10.1097/JSM.0b013e31819b51b3.

101. Bloomer RJ, Larson DE, Fisher-Wellman KH, Galpin AJ, Schilling BK. Effect of eicosapentaenoic and docosahexaenoic acid on resting and exercise-induced

inflammatory and oxidative stress biomarkers: a randomized, placebo controlled, cross-over study. Lipids Health Dis. 2009 Aug 19;8:36. doi: 10.1186/1476-511X-8-36.

102. Kiecolt-Glaser JK, Belury MA, Andridge R, Malarkey WB, Glaser R. Omega-3 supplementation lowers inflammation and anxiety in medical students: a randomized controlled trial. Brain Behav Immun. 2011 Nov;25(8):1725-34. doi: 10.1016/j.bbi.2011.07.229. Epub 2011 Jul 19.

103. Yusof HM, Miles EA, Calder P. Influence of very long-chain n-3 fatty acids on plasma markers of inflammation in middle-aged men. Prostaglandins Leukot Essent Fatty Acids. 2008 Mar;78(3):219-28. doi: 10.1016/j.plefa.2008.02.002. Epub 2008 Apr 9.

104. Kiecolt-Glaser JK, Belury MA, Andridge R, Malarkey WB, Glaser R. Omega-3 supplementation lowers inflammation and anxiety in medical students: a randomized controlled trial. Brain Behav Immun. 2011 Nov;25(8):1725-34. doi: 10.1016/j.bbi.2011.07.229. Epub 2011 Jul 19.

105. Ramel A, Martinez JA, Kiely M, Bandarra NM, Thorsdottir I. Moderate consumption of fatty fish reduces diastolic blood pressure in overweight and obese European young adults during energy restriction. Nutrition. 2010 Feb;26(2):168-74. doi: 10.1016/j.nut.2009.04.002. Epub 2009 May 31.

106. Campbell F, Dickinson HO, Critchley JA, Ford GA, Bradburn M. A systematic review of fish-oil supplements for the prevention and treatment of hypertension. Eur J Prev Cardiol. 2013 Feb;20(1):107-20. doi: 10.1177/2047487312437056. Epub 2012 Jan 30.

107. Nahas R, Sheikh O. Complementary and alternative medicine for the treatment of major depressive disorder. Can Fam Physician. 2011 Jun;57(6):659-63.

108. Sarris J, Mischoulon D, Schweitzer I. Omega-3 for bipolar disorder: meta-analyses of use in mania and bipolar depression. J Clin Psychiatry. 2012 Jan;73(1):81-6. doi: 10.4088/JCP.10r06710. Epub 2011 Aug 9.

109. Hamazaki T, Itomura M, Sawazaki S, Nagao Y. Anti-stress effects of DHA. Biofactors. 2000;13(1-4):41-5.

110. Sawazaki S, Hamazaki T, Yazawa K, Kobayashi M. The effect of docosahexaenoic acid on plasma catecholamine concentrations and glucose tolerance during long-lasting psychological stress: a double-blind placebo-controlled study. J Nutr Sci Vitaminol (Tokyo). 1999 Oct;45(5):655-65.

111. Lauretani F, Maggio M, Pizzarelli F, Michelassi S, Ruggiero C, Ceda GP, Bandinelli S, Ferrucci L. Omega-3 and renal function in older adults. Curr Pharm Des. 2009;15(36):4149-56.

112. De Caterina R, Madonna R, Massaro M. Effects of omega-3 fatty acids on cytokines and adhesion molecules. Curr Atheroscler Rep. 2004 Nov;6(6):485-91.

113. Simopoulos AP. The importance of the omega-6/omega-3 fatty acid ratio in cardiovascular disease and other chronic diseases. Exp Biol Med (Maywood). 2008 Jun;233(6):674-88. doi: 10.3181/0711-MR-311. Epub 2008 Apr 11.

114. Ka He, MD, MPH; Eric B. Rimm, ScD; Anwar Merchant, DMD, ScD; Bernard A. Rosner, PhD; Meir J. Stampfer, MD, DrPH; Walter C. Willett, MD, DrPH; Alberto Ascherio, MD, DrPH. Fish Consumption and Risk of Stroke in Men. JAMA.

2002;288(24):3130-3136. doi:10.1001/jama.288.24.3130.

115. Huang T, Bhulaidok S, Cai Z, Xu T, Xu F, Wahlqvist ML, Li D. Plasma phospholipids n-3 polyunsaturated fatty acid is associated with metabolic syndrome. Mol Nutr Food Res. 2010 Nov;54(11):1628-35. doi: 10.1002/mnfr.201000025.

116. Smith BK, Holloway GP, Reza-Lopez S, Jeram SM, Kang JX, Ma DW. A decreased n-6/n-3 ratio in the fat-1 mouse is associated with improved glucose tolerance. Appl Physiol Nutr Metab. 2010 Oct;35(5):699-706. doi: 10.1139/H10-066.

117. Rossi AS, Lombardo YB, Lacorte JM, Chicco AG, Rouault C, Slama G, Rizkalla SW. Dietary fish oil positively regulates plasma leptin and adiponectin levels in sucrose-fed, insulin-resistant rats. Am J Physiol Regul Integr Comp Physiol. 2005 Aug;289(2):R486-R494.

118. Huang T, Wahlqvist ML, Xu T, Xu A, Zhang A, Li D. Increased plasma n-3 polyunsaturated fatty acid is associated with improved insulin sensitivity in type 2 diabetes in China. Mol Nutr Food Res. 2010 May;54 Suppl 1:S112-9. doi: 10.1002/ mnfr.200900189.

119. Narendran R, Frankle WG, Mason NS, Muldoon MF, Moghaddam B (2012) Improved Working Memory but No Effect on Striatal Vesicular Monoamine Transporter Type 2 after Omega-3 Polyunsaturated Fatty Acid Supplementation. PLoS ONE 7(10): e46832. doi:10.1371/journal.pone.0046832.

120. Muldoon MF, Ryan CM, Sheu L, Yao JK, Conklin SM, Manuck SB. Serum phospholipid docosahexaenonic acid is associated with cognitive functioning during middle adulthood. J Nutr. 2010 Apr;140(4):848-53. doi: 10.3945/jn.109.119578. Epub 2010 Feb 24.

121. Chiu CC, Su KP, Cheng TC, Liu HC, Chang CJ, Dewey ME, Stewart R, Huang SY. The effects of omega-3 fatty acids monotherapy in Alzheimer's disease and mild cognitive impairment: a preliminary randomized double-blind placebo-controlled study. Prog Neuropsychopharmacol Biol Psychiatry. 2008 Aug 1;32(6):1538-44. doi: 10.1016/j.pnpbp.2008.05.015. Epub 2008 May 25.

122. Buckley JD, Howe PR. Anti-obesity effects of long-chain omega-3 polyunsaturated fatty acids. Obes Rev. 2009 Nov;10(6):648-59. doi: 10.1111/j.1467-789X.2009.00584.x. Epub 2009 May 12.

123. Cha SH, Fukushima A, Sakuma K, Kagawa Y. Chronic docosahexaenoic acid intake enhances expression of the gene for uncoupling protein 3 and affects pleiotropic mRNA levels in skeletal muscle of aged C57BL/6NJcl mice. J Nutr. 2001 Oct;131(10):2636-42.

124. Baillie RA, Takada R, Nakamura M, Clarke SD. Coordinate induction of peroxisomal acyl-CoA oxidase and UCP-3 by dietary fish oil: a mechanism for decreased body fat deposition. Prostaglandins Leukot Essent Fatty Acids. 1999 May-Jun;60(5-6):351-6.

125. Flachs P, Horakova O, Brauner P, Rossmeisl M, Pecina P, Franssen-van Hal N, Ruzickova J, Sponarova J, Drahota Z, Vlcek C, Keijer J, Houstek J, Kopecky J. Polyunsaturated fatty acids of marine origin upregulate mitochondrial biogenesis and induce beta-oxidation in white fat. Diabetologia. 2005 Nov;48(11):2365-75. Epub 2005 Oct 5.

126. Couet C, Delarue J, Ritz P, Antoine JM, Lamisse F. Effect of dietary fish oil on body fat

mass and basal fat oxidation in healthy adults. Int J Obes Relat Metab Disord. 1997 Aug;21(8):637-43.

127. Hessvik NP, Bakke SS, Fredriksson K, Boekschoten MV, Fjørkenstad A, Koster G, Hesselink MK, Kersten S, Kase ET, Rustan AC, Thoresen GH. Metabolic switching of human myotubes is improved by n-3 fatty acids. J Lipid Res. 2010 Aug;51(8):2090-104. doi: 10.1194/jlr.M003319. Epub 2010 Apr 2.

128. Mogelson S, Pieper SJ, Lange LG. Thermodynamic bases for fatty acid ethyl ester synthase catalyzed esterification of free fatty acid with ethanol and accumulation of fatty acid ethyl esters. Biochemistry. 1984 Aug 28;23(18):4082-7.

129. Beckermann B, Beneke M, Seitz I. Comparative bioavailability of eicosapentaenoic acid and docasahexaenoic acid from triglycerides, free fatty acids and ethyl esters in volunteers. Arzneimittelforschung. 1990 Jun;40(6):700-4.

130. Dyerberg J, Madsen P, Møller JM, Aardestrup I, Schmidt EB. Bioavailability of marine n-3 fatty acid formulations. Prostaglandins Leukot Essent Fatty Acids. 2010 Sep;83(3):137-41. doi: 10.1016/j.plefa.2010.06.007.

131. Neubronner J, Schuchardt JP, Kressel G, Merkel M, von Schacky C, Hahn A. Enhanced increase of omega-3 index in response to long-term n-3 fatty acid supplementation from triacylglycerides versus ethyl esters. Eur J Clin Nutr. 2011 Feb;65(2):247-54. doi: 10.1038/ejcn.2010.239. Epub 2010 Nov 10.

132. Yang LY, Kuksis A, Myher JJ. Lipolysis of menhaden oil triacylglycerols and the corresponding fatty acid alkyl esters by pancreatic lipase in vitro: a reexamination. J Lipid Res. 1990 Jan;31(1):137-47.

133. Best CA, Laposata M. Fatty acid ethyl esters: toxic non-oxidative metabolites of ethanol and markers of ethanol intake. Front Biosci. 2003 Jan 1;8:e202-17.

134. Haber PS, Wilson JS, Apte MV, Pirola RC. Fatty acid ethyl esters increase rat pancreatic lysosomal fragility. J Lab Clin Med. 1993 Jun;121(6):759-64.

135. Yuan GJ, Zhou XR, Gong ZJ, Zhang P, Sun XM, Zheng SH. Expression and activity of inducible nitric oxide synthase and endothelial nitric oxide synthase correlate with ethanol-induced liver injury. World J Gastroenterol. 2006 Apr 21;12(15):2375-81.

136. Laposata EA, Lange LG. Presence of nonoxidative ethanol metabolism in human organs commonly damaged by ethanol abuse. Science. 1986 Jan 31;231(4737):497-9.

137. Werner J, Laposata M, Fernández-del Castillo C, Saghir M, Iozzo RV, Lewandrowski KB, Warshaw AL. Pancreatic injury in rats induced by fatty acid ethyl ester, a nonoxidative metabolite of alcohol. Gastroenterology. 1997 Jul;113(1):286-94.

138. Foran SE, Flood JG, Lewandrowski KB. Measurement of mercury levels in concentrated over-the-counter fish oil preparations: is fish oil healthier than fish? Arch Pathol Lab Med. 2003 Dec;127(12):1603-5.

139. Marit Aursand, Revilija Mozuraityte, Kristin Hamre, Helle Knutsen, Amund Maage, Augustine Arukwe. Description of the processes in the value chain and risk assessment of decomposition substances and oxidation products in fish oils.

140. Schaller JL. Mercury and fish oil supplements. MedGenMed. 2001 Apr 13;3(2):20.

141. Melanson SF, Lewandrowski EL, Flood JG, Lewandrowski KB. Measurement of

organochlorines in commercial over-the-counter fish oil preparations: implications for dietary and therapeutic recommendations for omega-3 fatty acids and a review of the literature. Arch Pathol Lab Med. 2005 Jan;129(1):74-7.

142. Moore DR, Robinson MJ, Fry JL, Tang JE, Glover EI, Wilkinson SB, Prior T, Tarnopolsky MA, Phillips SM. Ingested protein dose response of muscle and albumin protein synthesis after resistance exercise in young men. Am J Clin Nutr. 2009 Jan;89(1):161-8. doi: 10.3945/ajcn.2008.26401. Epub 2008 Dec 3.

143. Yang Y, Breen L, Burd NA, Hector AJ, Churchward-Venne TA, Josse AR, Tarnopolsky MA, Phillips SM. Resistance exercise enhances myofibrillar protein synthesis with graded intakes of whey protein in older men. Br J Nutr. 2012 Nov 28;108(10):1780-8. doi: 10.1017/S0007114511007422. Epub 2012 Feb 7.

144. Pennings B, Groen B, de Lange A, Gijsen AP, Zorenc AH, Senden JM, van Loon LJ. Amino acid absorption and subsequent muscle protein accretion following graded intakes of whey protein in elderly men. Am J Physiol Endocrinol Metab. 2012 Apr 15;302(8):E992-9. doi: 10.1152/ajpendo.00517.2011. Epub 2012 Feb 14.

145. Nosaka K, Sacco P, Mawatari K. Effects of amino acid supplementation on muscle soreness and damage. Int J Sport Nutr Exerc Metab. 2006 Dec;16(6):620-35.

146. Bemben MG, Lamont HS. Creatine supplementation and exercise performance: recent findings. Sports Med. 2005;35(2):107-25.

147. Kreider RB. Effects of creatine supplementation on performance and training adaptations. Mol Cell Biochem. 2003 Feb;244(1-2):89-94.

148. Preen D, Dawson B, Goodman C, Beilby J, Ching S. Creatine supplementation: a comparison of loading and maintenance protocols on creatine uptake by human skeletal muscle. Int J Sport Nutr Exerc Metab. 2003 Mar;13(1):97-111.

149. Green AL, Hultman E, Macdonald IA, Sewell DA, Greenhaff PL. Carbohydrate ingestion augments skeletal muscle creatine accumulation during creatine supplementation in humans. Am J Physiol. 1996 Nov;271(5 Pt 1):E821-6.

150. Bassini-Cameron A, Monteiro A, Gomes A, Werneck-de-Castro JP, Cameron L. Glutamine protects against increases in blood ammonia in football players in an exercise intensity-dependent way. Br J Sports Med. 2008 Apr;42(4):260-6. Epub 2007 Nov 5.

151. Gleeson M. Dosing and efficacy of glutamine supplementation in human exercise and sport training. J Nutr. 2008 Oct;138(10):2045S-2049S.

152 Hoffman JR, Ratamess NA, Kang J, Rashti SL, Kelly N, Gonzalez AM, Stec M, Anderson S, Bailey BL, Yamamoto LM, Hom LL, Kupchak BR, Faigenbaum AD, Maresh CM. Examination of the efficacy of acute L-alanyl-L-glutamine ingestion during hydration stress in endurance exercise. J Int Soc Sports Nutr. 2010 Feb 3;7:8. doi: 10.1186/1550-2783-7-8.

153. Hibbeln JR, Nieminen LR, Blasbalg TL, Riggs JA, Lands WE. Healthy intakes of n-3 and n-6 fatty acids: estimations considering worldwide diversity. Am J Clin Nutr. 2006 Jun;83(6 Suppl):1483S-1493S.

154. Artemis P. Simopoulos, MD, Alexander Leaf, MD and Norman Salem Jr, PhD. Workshop on the Essentiality of and Recommended Dietary Intakes for Omega-6 and Omega-3 Fatty Acids. J Am Coll Nutr October 1999 vol. 18 no. 5 487-489.

INDEX

Printed in Great Britain
by Amazon.co.uk, Ltd.,
Marston Gate.